YO-BUT-342

The Rights
of the
Pregnant
Parent

Revised Edition

Valmai
Howe
Elkins

Schocken Books • New York

First published by Schocken Books 1980
10 9 8 7 6 5 4 3 2 1   80 81 82 83

Copyright © 1976 by Valmai Howe Elkins

Library of Congress Cataloging in Publication Data

Elkins, Valmai Howe.
    The rights of the pregnant parent.
    Originally published by Waxwing Productions, Toronto,
    Ont. and Two Continents, New York.
    Bibliography: p.
    Includes index.
    1. Natural childbirth. 2. Hospitals, Gynecologic and ob-
stetric. I. Title. (DNLM: 1. Labor. 2. Natural childbirth.
WQ150 E43r)
RG661.E44 1980   618.4'5   80-14828

Printed in the United States of America.
This edition is not for sale in Canada.

2216700

For David and Tilke.

Acknowledgments

I deeply appreciate the help of the people who aided me in my research for this book by sharing with me their time and knowledge — Dr. Pierre Vellay and the staff of the Château Belvedere, Paris; Prof. Treffer and the maternity staff of the Wilhemina Gasthuis, Amsterdam; Dr. Jan Kleinhout and the maternity staff of the University Hospital of Amsterdam; Nancy Fox-Martin, Lamaze instructor, and Neliek and Sybren DeJeu, Amsterdam; Billie Carlston, R.N., Manchester Memorial Hospital, Manchester, Connecticut; and Chloe Fisher, S.R.N., of Oxford, England.

My warmest thanks to Montreal obstetrician David Rhea for his encouragement and support over the past nine years, and to Elisabeth Bing and Murray Enkin for their inspiration and enthusiasm.

My thanks to the executive committees, past and present, of the Montreal Childbirth Education Association, for their unselfish work to promote Prepared Childbirth; and to the hundreds of men and women from my classes who have generously shared their experiences, emotions and ideas with me, and who provided a great deal of the material in this book. And to Nicole and Bill Abbott — who cheerfully agreed to be photographed for the front cover of this book, shortly before the birth of their daughter, Genevieve.

My sincere thanks to Bonnie Buxton, whose constant enthusiasm, insight and help far exceeded the normal bounds as editor and publisher.

Finally, my loving thanks to my family — my parents, my brother Dr. Arthur Howe and his wife Katy for their encouragement; to Vivian Elkins, the late Stuart Elkins and to "Plim" Plimley for constant help. And most of all, to David and Tilke, whose understanding, patience and love made it possible for me to write the book.

Contents

Foreword

Psychoprophylaxis did not begin with a concern for parents' rights. It began with a concern for tools — tools to enable women to cope with labor, to work with their uterine contractions. Tools to help them obtain relief from the agony of the unmedicated, unsupported childbirth practices of Europe, and to manage without the massive medication which rendered them helpless in North America. Those of us who were teaching Lamaze techniques in the early years after their introduction were concerned only with the refinement and improvement of those techniques. We did not and could not realize at that time, how their widespread utilization would have ramifications infinitely more important than the relatively minor effects for which they were intended.

As women became more aware of their own bodies, and their own ability to actively participate in the birth of their child, they became aware that this was not enough. Their consciousness was raised. They began to realize that the care they were receiving was given by a benign dictatorship, and it was not necessarily the care they wished to receive. They wanted to participate, not only in the labor, but in the management as well.

This increasing awareness by the care-receiver was bound to have an effect on the care-givers as well. When the patient was no longer a passive recipient of their well-intentioned ministrations, the physician or nurse felt slighted, unappreciated, threatened, and angry.

Women approached the health team with a chip on their shoulders because of their stereotyped picture of the inflexible medical establishment. Doctors and nurses reacted to their own stereotype of a demanding and unreasonable patient. It was confrontation rather than communication. Instead of the enemy being the potential hazards of childbirth, those who should have been the allies became the antagonists.

Anger and accusations are obviously not the answer. The obstetrical team is concerned with the welfare of the mother, the child and the family. The family is equally concerned with their health and safety. They wish this safety without, however, losing their dignity as human beings, or their ability to express their love and joy in the emotionally overwhelming experience of giving birth.

Books have been written criticizing the medical establishment; some factual, some bitter, some outraged. They are important, because they vividly bring the conflict to our attention. But they do not help to solve the impasse. This book is the first to attempt to do so.

It seems right to us that this book was written by Valmai Elkins. We have known her since she first became involved in childbirth education. She showed herself from the start to be dedicated, enquiring, and innovative. She is outspoken, yet soft spoken, persevering and determined yet warm and sensitive.

It is, therefore, no surprise that in this book she has shown both sides how the deadlock can be broken, how dialogue can be started and continued. This book could not have been written 10 years ago. Both sides were too polarized to see another point of view. Time and maturity have made the professional ready to listen, and the consumer aware that there can be communication without capitulation.

We are grateful that this book has been written. It should be read by parents and professionals alike.

Elisabeth Bing
Clinical Assistant Professor
Department of Obstetrics and Gynecology
New York Medical College

Murray Enkin, M.D., F.R.C.S. (C)
Associate Professor of Obstetrics and Gynecology
McMaster University
Hamilton, Ontario

Introduction

The doctor who cared for me during the birth of my first child was very skeptical about Prepared Childbirth. Because it was my first baby, I was content to go along with his wish to induce labor, even though I was not overdue. (Wednesday was "his" day at the hospital we'd chosen.)

I also submitted to an epidural and episiotomy. Somehow my husband and I managed to keep up with the breathing techniques we'd learned. . .

When I finally became pregnant again last summer, I returned to the same doctor. As the months went by, I became increasingly aware of a difference in philosophy between the doctor and me. He wasn't willing to let me try a vaginal delivery without an epidural and forceps. He refused to discuss "allowing" my husband to accompany for a Caesarean under local anesthetic, should that procedure prove necessary. In fact, he laughed at me when I brought up the subject, although my first baby had nearly been Caesarean.

A friend had lent me your book in early pregnancy. The more I read it, the more I realized that we were being cheated of an important life-experience.

Finally, two weeks before my due date, I re-read your words, "Remember — if you are changing doctors, the sooner, the better. But it is better to change doctors late than compromise yourselves in what can be a beautiful shared experience." The next day, I phoned a doctor recommended to me by our Lamaze instructor. What a difference!

The requests which were denied at the first hospital were

*routine at the second hospital. The nurses were familiar with
Prepared Childbirth and were most supportive. No one urged
me to take medication, and everyone was most understanding
when I declined.*

*My husband was able to accompany me from the labor
room directly to the delivery. He and two nurses coached me
until the doctor arrived.*

*Feeling the baby leave my body was one of the most incred-
ible experiences in my life. What a shock when we found he
was ten pounds one ounce! We had accomplished what the
first doctor seemed to find impossible, reactionary and laughable. We had worked together, in dignity and peace to bring
forth this new person who would share our lives.*

*At the first hospital, my daughter and I were separated for
nearly twenty-four hours while I became more frantic and uncomfortable. This time, we were able to be together in the
recovery room for an hour while the baby and I were bathed
and he was put to the breast. . .*

*Thank you for the part your book played in making
David's arrival so exciting and moving an experience.*

— Marion Holmes

I first wrote this book because each year thousands of
North American parents were frustrated in their attempts at a
positive birth experience. I was saddened and angered by the
hundreds of complaints I received from both women and men
— both prepared and unprepared — who felt that they had
been cheated of a beautiful, shared childbirth.

Admittedly, it's a biased book. My opinions are based on
the thirteen years I have spent as a childbirth educator, observing hundreds of births, coaching many women through
childbirth, instructing thousands of couples in prepared childbirth techniques, listening to their postnatal comments — as
well as my own experience as a woman in childbirth.

This experience, coupled with an ever-growing body of

scientific literature on human birth, has convinced me that the simplest, least medicated method of childbirth is normally best for mother and infant — and for the father as well. (By childbirth, I include labor, delivery and the hospital stay of mother and baby.)

Some people have asked why I've entitled this book, *The Rights of the Pregnant Parent* — rather than The Rights of the Pregnant Woman. I chose the former title because more men are becoming involved in parenthood than ever before. For most couples today, children are not just an accident. They're the result of a conscious decision on the part of both the woman and her mate. And once the decision has been made to have a baby, an increasing number of men want to participate in both the childbirth experience and the child-raising process. Or as one young male client told me, "I want to do the thing *right.*"

Many how-to books have been written about the revolutionary method of Prepared Childbirth, sometimes called the Lamaze Method. In this method, the woman conditions herself to participate actively in labor and delivery with the help of a coach (usually the baby's father). Usually, medication is not necessary; this method considerably reduces the discomfort of childbirth.

Recently, other books have been written questioning the traditional birth practices on this continent, deploring the depersonalization and mechanization of "birthing." Some of these books have advocated a return to home birth or the renaissance of the midwife.

Yet even with a superb home birth system, not all women can birth safely at home: there are advances in obstetrical care for "high-risk" babies and mothers, which home birth cannot provide. But I firmly believe that Prepared Childbirth is the *only* way to deliver a child. "But what if it's an abnormal birth?" some critics of the method may ask. The fact is that about 90% of births are normal — and made easier, and in some cases pain-free by this method. Even a high-risk or abnormal birth becomes less traumatic — both physically and emotionally — if the woman and her mate are prepared for labor and delivery.

Since the first edition of this book in 1977, there have been changes in birth on this continent — brought about by concerned parents and professionals. Childbirth education programs have mushroomed; hospital policies have become more flexible. There is growing support for parents who seek alternatives in childbirth; stronger focus on the emotional needs of the new family; and improved communication between parents and staff.

But unfortunately, the birthing practices in North America are increasingly geared to the high-risk case rather than to the normal one. As "actively managed" childbirth becomes the norm, there is a dramatic increase in the Caesarean birth rate — from 4-6% in 1974 to a current 12-15%. Indeed, at many hospitals I have visited, the rate runs as high as 20-30%! While few would deny the value of the Caesarean procedure in certain high-risk situations, I feel we must examine very carefully a birthing system which may soon require 20-30% of pregnant women to give birth by major surgery.

However, I believe that the picture is not so gloomy as some critics have charged. You *can* have the childbirth you choose, within the hospital setting, if you have the tools to work within the system. The tools are information, conviction, tact — and a community which backs you up in your demands.

These tools are crucial — on this continent where most hospitals view childbirth as an illness, and many medical personnel still tend to discourage, interrupt or thwart even the prepared couple in their attempt to have a shared, non-medicated childbirth. At least three or four times a week, somebody phones me to relate a hospital incident which caused unnecessary discomfort or anxiety during the stressful period of labor, birth and the days immediately following. The complaints range from non-communication of staff members to denial of choices in birth to cases of gross obstetrical mismanagement.

Traumatic experience or joyous event? What are the chances of each? Is there any way of knowing what it will be? What steps can be taken in advance to make sure that you have the type of birth experience of your choice, whether it is the Lamaze or any other method?

Knowing the childbirth techniques is extremely important. Equally important is the conviction that as a pregnant parent you have rights — coupled with a refusal to take No for an answer. The right to have classes available in a particular method, or to have the father present at the delivery are only two aspects. Equally important is the right to have available all of the essentials for a healthy baby and the positive emotional growth of the family.

As a result of my experience with thousands of couples, I have defined what I consider to be the rights of every pregnant woman and her partner. These are basic human rights. Unfortunately, at this time, none has been legally defined.

1. The right to a supportive doctor.
2. The right to a healthy baby.
3. The right to childbirth education.
4. The right to a shared birth experience.
5. The right to childbirth with dignity.
6. The right to family-centered maternity care.

In the following chapters I will examine these rights more closely and suggest techniques in communicating with doctors and hospital staff to get the childbirth you want. I will also take a critical look at traditional North American obstetrical methods, comparing them with the systems in countries where Prepared Childbirth is the norm. Finally I will conclude by outlining some methods by which couples, the medical profession and the medical community at large, can improve the North American way of birth.

I must emphasize that, although I firmly believe that these rights should be available, whether or not they are exercised is entirely up to the individual. They are "rights" and not "rules" — to be taken advantage of if the woman and man wish; to be left unused if that's their decision.

One more thing. With rights come responsibilities. If you decide to pursue these rights you automatically assume some responsibility for the care given (or withheld). To bypass routines — at present almost unavoidable to put these rights into effect — you must be aware of any consequences which may result. For example, if the woman chooses to avoid an enema in early labor, she takes responsibility for any unfortunate side-effects! Although such side-effects may be highly unlikely, a decision *not* to follow traditional hospital routines should not be taken lightly.

Unfortunately many doctors think of couples who wish to exercise choice in their childbirth experience, in terms of the word "demand". As you'll discover in the following chapters, demanding is not taken too well by the medical profession. It is easier and more effective to discuss and communicate rather than demand.

Furthermore, to many doctors, "demand" is closely allied to "fad". The couple who demand something unconventional without taking the trouble to research it or discuss it may be labelled "faddists" by the doctor — damaging the reception for those responsible couples who have become well-informed before requesting something out of the mainstream.

I write from the point of view of a physiotherapist and childbirth educator. My concern is for parents and babies rather than for smoothly running obstetrical departments — a view that may clash with those conservative members of the medical profession who still adhere to the "Doctor is King" philosophy. Fortunately, not all obstetricians and nursing personnel are rigid and inflexible: many are open to new ideas, providing they are discussed beforehand. So perhaps this is a good place to thank the numbers of doctors and nurses who have encouraged my clients and me in our efforts towards more fulfilling childbirth. Some of these medical people at first viewed us as faddists — but their skepticism has turned to support and in many cases to deeply rooted conversion to our cause.

It's possible to turn an "ordinary" birth into a time of exhilaration and achievement, without rejecting the advantages a modern hospital can provide. But to do so, you need the following elements: solid understanding of the birth process and the ability to work with it; the support of someone you love and who loves you; and a knowledge of your rights in childbirth — plus the determination to stand up for them. These are the elements of a method which takes Prepared Childbirth one step further: I call it Ultra-Prepared Childbirth (UPC). This is the story of hundreds of couples who have used UPC to make the current obstetrical system work for them — couples who remember the births of their children as precious and unforgettable moments, symbolic of a rich, intimate and growing love relationship.

My husband, David, and I share such memories. In 1973, he coached as I pushed my daughter Tilke into the world. Her birth was easy, ecstatic, non-medicated and accomplished with no interference and very little pain.

With this book, I wish your yet-to-be born child an equally joyous birth.

                                        VALMAI HOWE ELKINS

1 In search of a better birth

Our so-called traditional childbirth practices are predicated on three fascinating myths. The first is that pregnancy is a disease. Pregnant women go to doctors; doctors treat disease; therefore pregnancy is a disease.

The second myth is that doctors deliver babies. Doctors don't deliver babies, women do. But when the myth is accepted, doctors feel they have to carry out their part of the contract. The doctor replaces the parents as the star in the drama of birth, and patterns of interference in birthing are inevitable.

The third myth is that all mothers are virgins. Because of this myth we have kept husbands out of labor rooms and delivery rooms, even examining rooms for fear of shocking him, or her.''

—*Dr. Murray Enkin, obstetrician.*

You are a pregnant woman in early labor. The contractions are coming close together with increasing intensity. You leave your home and drive with your mate to a large hospital, presenting yourselves at the admission desk. A nurse escorts you to a labor room, a small cubicle containing little more than a bed. You exchange your street clothes for a short gown, and climb onto the bed. The nurse takes your blood pressure, temperature and respiration and listens to your baby's heart rate. (Meanwhile, your mate waits anxiously in the fathers' waiting room until he is permitted to join you — maybe 45 minutes later.)

"Lie down, please" says the nurse crisply. She shaves your lower pubic hair; contractions are coming more frequently, and you try, without much success, to relax. Now she asks you to lie on your side for an enema. "Hold it in for a few moments," she tells you — just as you have a contraction. Through the pain you dimly remember being taught how to relax and breathe during contractions — but how can you relax and "hold it in" at the same time?

You go to the washroom to expel the enema. You clutch at the doorknob and bite your lip as another contraction rolls over you: if only your mate were here! Twenty minutes later an intravenous tube is inserted into the vein of your arm, attached to a bottle on a stand by the bedside. "You musn't eat anything," the nurse cautions. "But this will give you energy — and it keeps a vein open just in case there's an emergency." While you're imagining dire emergencies, a belt with a fetal heart rate attachment is strapped around your abdomen. "This will record the heart beat for the next hours of labor," the nurse says, and leaves the room.

An intern enters with a sheaf of papers and starts asking for detailed information about your family's medical history and your pregnancy. You try to remember where your mother was born but the contractions are coming thick and fast. You try to find a comfortable position — impossible without disturbing the IV or monitor. Just then the nurse pops in and suggests a shot of medication "to take the edge off things."

A resident doctor enters, feels your abdomen and asks you to lie flat, bring your knees up and let them fall apart. He

examines you vaginally to measure progress of labor. Finally
your mate returns, hovering over the bed, taking care to avoid
the IV and monitor. But each time a doctor enters, he'll be
asked to step outside.

Contractions become more intense. The nurse says it's time
for the local anesthetic. You may have planned to have a non-
medicated birth, but you're tired, uncomfortable and
irritable. "Most women need one," the nurse tells you.
"Don't feel disappointed if you need something." You
readily agree.

Your mate leaves for the waiting room. You're wheeled into the bright, cold delivery room. Gleaming steel cabinets
containing equipment line the walls; tubes for general
anesthetic run from floor to ceiling at the head of a short,
narrow table in the centre of the room. You're asked to sit
over the edge of the table. An anesthetist paints the lower part
of your back with ice-cold antiseptic and injects local
anesthesia into the lower back. A nurse checks your blood
pressure. You're wheeled back to your room. Everything
seems to have stopped.

You doze off and when you awake a nurse is adjusting the
IV bottle. Soon contractions become stronger and you're
wheeled into the delivery room. If your doctor is "advanced", your mate changes into special clothing to accompany you; otherwise, he leaves for the waiting room. For
some reason your own doctor is not there.

You wriggle across onto the delivery table, your legs
strangely heavy from the anesthetic. A nurse raises your legs
into padded stirrups, which hold them wide apart. Your legs
and abdomen are draped with sterile sheets. "Push!" says
someone through the fog.

"I can't," you moan. It all seems so...hard. After what
seems like hours, you're given a shot of local anesthetic, so
that you can't feel the doctor's scalpel as it slices below your
vagina, in what is known as episiotomy.

"Push!" someone says again, while the doctor uses forceps
to bring the baby out.

"It's a girl!" he says, and you'd love to touch her, but your hands are strapped to the sides of the table in leather thongs. Just then, you're given a shot in the arm to hasten the expulsion of the placenta. More contractions; within ten minutes it's out. Your daughter's cord was clamped and cut within a minute of her birth. She's now in an incubator at the side of the room, having been identified, weighed and silver nitrate solution placed in her eyes to prevent infection.

The doctor repairs your episiotomy, leaving the minute he finishes the last stitch. You cuddle your baby briefly before she's wheeled off to the nursery. You're then wheeled to a "recovery area" and given a shot for possible pain. Your mate stays with you for an hour, then goes home. Exhausted, you slip into a drugged sleep.

Under the bright lights of a central nursery, your baby lies in her little glass-sided crib, one more baby in a row of other newborns. She has the strong sucking reflex with which all newborns are born, but there is nothing to suck — her lips press together futilely. The warmth and shadows of the uterus, the rocking of your body are suddenly replaced by artificial warmth; a person is replaced with efficient objects. When she cries, she will be given a bottle of glucose and water to suck, then returned to her crib until she is checked by the pediatrician and pronounced "ready" to be shown to you. Her contact with you will be regulated, her feedings given by a bottle. If you try to breastfeed her, the feedings will be carefully recorded and you will probably be encouraged to improve on nature — with supplementary bottles.

After three to five days, you and your baby return home. You, your mate and your baby have just experienced a "normal" birth — as it is managed in most North American hospitals today.

I watched my first North American birth in 1967. I had just turned twenty and was fresh from the Melbourne School of Physiotherapy in Australia. I was horrified. During my training I had watched various births, but the management of birth in that small community hospital struck me as positively sadistic. I had not seen stirrups or handcuffs before — instinctively I shrank from them. Nor had I seen episiotomy, and the seeming necessity to perform surgery on every woman who gave birth perplexed me.

In those days, Australia used the British method of childbirth developed by Dr. Grantly Dick-Read and made popular after World War II. The woman in late labor "bore down" while lying on her back in a somewhat curled position, supporting her own bent legs on her chest. As soon as the baby's head crowned, she would roll onto her side ("Sims' Position"), with her back slightly bent, and the attendant would support the upper leg while the baby was eased out. In this position, there was less pressure on the perineum, and episiotomy was usually not necessary. And unlike the flat-on-back, draped and shackled North American position, Sims' Position enabled the mother to watch the entire delivery. I remember the nurse cheerfully telling the women, "Now look between your legs and you'll see your baby's head."

After asking questions of the Ontario hospital's nursing staff, I discovered that I hadn't stumbled into a barbaric outpost after all — that what I was viewing was the North American way of birth as it generally occurs. I later learned that some hospitals have modified some practices, and there are small variations depending on the state of enlightenment of the chief of obstetrics. But for the most part, the Canadian or American woman delivers her child while lying flat on her back, legs in the air — working against gravity and needing all the help that the obstetrician with his anesthetic, scalpel and forceps can give, thankful for any drug which can take away the pain. I vowed to a colleague that if this was what women went through I would never have a baby!

I could scarcely have predicted that a few years later, not only would I have become a childbirth educator who had prepared thousands of women and men for childbirth — but a mother as well. In 1970, I had married David Elkins, and in 1973 using the tools of Prepared Childbirth which I had been teaching, we became parents — together. Our enthusiasm over the shared, non-medicated and somewhat unorthodox birth of our daughter convinced us that most North American couples are cheated by obstetrical "management."

My search for an alternative to the managed birth of the North American hospital eventually took me to maternity hospitals in France and Holland. I wanted to see the French "Lamaze" method of childbirth in its native form, and the Dutch way of birth interested me on several counts. Holland is notable because of its low neonatal death rate — it ranks only slightly behind Sweden, the lowest — and because it is a country which offers excellent systems and care for both home and hospital birth. Doris Haire, past president of the International Childbirth Education Association, had spoken of birth in The Netherlands in glowing terms at a conference which I had attended in 1972. In December of 1974, David and I decided to investigate firsthand. The following birth is typical of the ones I witnessed in Amsterdam.

Childbirth in the Netherlands

Sophie R., 25, expecting her first child, arrived at the old, rambling Wilhemina Gasthuis, one of Amsterdam's older general hospitals, late in the afternoon. The large, eighty bed maternity unit is friendly, the staff relaxed. Sophie and her husband entered a modest cubicle which contained what seemed an ordinary hospital bed, a small table and an easy chair.

After she had changed into a short gown, a midwife listened to the baby's heartbeat with a simple fetal stethoscope and examined her internally. Her cervix was already three centimeters dilated. Admission forms had been completed at an earlier date via her doctor's office. Sophie was not given a shave — the doctor believed it unnecessary. Because labor was moving quite rapidly she was not given an enema.

As the contractions increased in intensity, Sophie breathed along with them. Her husband never left her side. Occasionally, the midwife checked in and encouraged them, bringing Sophie a bowl of soup shortly after her arrival at the hospital. When Sophie began to feel the urge to push, the doctor came into the cubicle and examined her. Yes, she could begin. Midwife and doctor stood by while Sophie lifted and supported her legs while her husband lifted her shoulders. Nothing was said. Sophie continued to push in an atmosphere of perfect calm. When the first dark wet hairs appeared at the opening, the doctor applied counter-pressure with a sterile pad to the bulging perineum and whispered to her to pant. The head rose, the face burst out, the doctor rotated and eased the shoulders out, then held the child, a pink healthy girl, up for its mother. She touched her daughter before the cord was clamped. The baby was placed on her side between Sophie's legs and mucous was sucked out of nose and mouth. The doctor massaged the tiny back, and the cry was healthy and strong — but there was almost no more crying. After a few minutes, the cord was cut, the child was wrapped in a warm blanket and passed to the mother.Mother and father embraced.

The only sterile things in the room had been the doctor's gloves and the sterile pads applied to the perineum. The father wore regular street clothes. Sophie was not draped. There were no stirrups. There was no spotlight as the child emerged, and no noise. No episiotomy was performed and there was not even the smallest tearing of the perineum. No medication had been used.

Baby Anita was then taken to an observation area in the centre of the room outside the curtain which made Sophie's cubicle private. The curtain was drawn back: the baby was placed in a small crib, attached to eight others in rows of three under a soft light. There, the pediatrician examined her while the parents watched. All was well. Mother, father and baby went to the hospital room together and mother and baby would not be separated during the hospital stay. The placenta came away about 30 minutes after birth, and a nurse brought the parents cups of tea. Outside, the Amsterdam twilight fell,

and from an adjoining room came the cry of another
newborn. Then all was calm.

I watched several births at this hospital and was greatly impressed by the calm, unhurried atmosphere; the wonderful
verbal support of the midwives. At the older hospitals in the
city, maternity staff are mostly trained midwives who manage
the labor and do internal exams before the doctor delivers. By
North American standards, facilities are modest — simple
cubicles, which are used for both labor and delivery. The beds
can be quickly converted into a fairly conventional delivery
table by removing the lower section and attaching stirrups.
This conversion is rarely needed — only in fewer than 5% of
cases, where forceps are necessary.

"In this country childbirth is viewed as a normal part of
life," Dr. Treffer, Associate Professor of Obstetrics at this
hospital told me, an opinion which I was to hear constantly
during my Dutch visit. Dutch statistics are impressive.
Holland vies only with Sweden for the lowest infant mortality
rate in the world, with 11.4 infant deaths per 1,000 live births
in 1972 (.3 higher than Sweden). Canada was eleventh, at
17.1, and the U.S.A. nineteenth at 18.5 deaths per 1,000.[1]

Back in Montreal, I spoke at a meeting of case room and
obstetrical nurses and showed them the slides which I had
been able to make of a Dutch birth. At first the reaction was,
"It looks so terribly *unprofessional* . . . no draping, no
stirrups!" After a discussion, however, many nurses saw advantages to such a low-key birthing.

Later, in the fall of 1975, David and I spoke at a large U.S.
hospital which prides itself on its "family-centered"
attitudes. Our presentation was for nursing personnel and
their partners. As the first slide appeared, one nurse whispered audibly to her mate, "Oh my God, I don't believe it —
don't look dear." One case room nurse joked about our slides
as pornographic: the concept of a normal "unmanaged"
birth seemed to be entirely unacceptable to her.

Let's compare statistics. There are some amazing differences, not easily dismissed by national characteristics.

	CANADA	U.S.	HOLLAND
Infant mortality rate	17.1*	18.5	11.4
Women prepared for birth	less than 50%	less than 50%	more than 80%
Obstetrical medication	85%	85%	2-5%
Forceps deliveries	60%	60%	5%
Inductions	15-20%	15-20%	5%
Episiotomy	more than 80%	more than 80%	15-20%
Caesarean Section	8%	8%	2%[2]

Across the Netherlands about 60% of births occur at home. In the cities about 60% occur in hospital. For low-risk women there is free choice between home or hospital. Each choice is backed by excellent prenatal care and medical back-up.

Dr. Jan Kleinhout of the obstetrical department at the Free Academic (University) Hospital of Amsterdam agreed with Prof. Treffer. "Birth is a family affair here. Most births are attended by a general practitioner or midwife. We've never had to go through a 'natural childbirth' movement here because it's always been this way. We regard childbirth as a normal physiological event. We don't interfere with normal birth and at this hospital we use drugs in only 2% of cases. Most women are trained in some form of breathing and relaxation. We believe that verbal sedation is better than drugs, but in this country we are more cautious of drugs. Look at the average North American bathroom cabinet — full of drugs! You don't find that here."

I asked why he thought the infant mortality rate for the Netherlands is so low. "We screen high-risk pregnancy very carefully. Women planning to have their babies at home see a midwife regularly and an obstetrician once during pregnancy. All high-risk cases give birth in a hospital with an obstetrician. And we don't interfere with normal labor. It is not good to interfere."

I was shown around the maternity unit of the University Hospital of Amsterdam and saw labor-delivery rooms similar to those at the Wilhemina Gasthuis — perhaps a little more

*deaths per 1,000 live births.

spacious and elaborate — along with a similarly designed central infant examining area.

I viewed all the latest equipment for high-risk cases: it's all there but I was told it's rarely needed. "We did introduce fetal monitors for low-risk births, but they were withdrawn because we noticed that staff were paying more attention to the equipment than to the women," one doctor told me. "Now we monitor only the high-risk cases in this way."

There seemed to be no private rooms in the maternity section — only three-bed rooms with small adjoining glass partitioned nurseries. Babies stay with their mothers all day and go into the little nursery at night, where the mother can have easy access to her baby, under the supervision of a nurse. Young children may visit their mothers, and the atmosphere here was as informal as the birthing area.

In one room I noticed a nurse feeding a baby milk from a tiny spoon while the mother watched. I asked why spoon feeding was used. "This baby needs some supplement to her mother's milk, but we do not use a bottle because the difference between breast and bottle feeding can confuse the baby and weaken the sucking at the breast," the nurse replied.

Nancy Fox-Martin is one of the few Lamaze instructors in Amsterdam. She told me of her preparation for birth in New York with Elisabeth Bing, her growing interest and her training to teach Lamaze. The Dutch have their own "method" of childbirth preparation which although extremely effective is difficult to categorize. Nancy works at the Central Israel Ziekenverpleging assisting at births. She teaches couples the Lamaze method in her home and often coaches them in labor as well. "The CIZ has a very small maternity unit — only 14 beds," Nancy told me, "We try to make it as much like home as possible. The couple are never separated. Admission procedures are all taken care of before they arrive at the hospital. Women can move around freely and eat and drink lightly. Shaves and enemas are assessed strictly on an individual basis. Some doctors prefer a shave;

others will ask the woman to give herself a "crew-cut" with manicure scissors if she is opposed to a shave. If she has had a bowel movement at home we don't think an enema is necessary. If her cervix is more than four centimeters dilated we never give one. When we do we use only a small one to empty the lower part of the rectum." She handed me a tiny tube marked "Microlax" — beside this the routine North American "Fleet" enema looks like an enema for an elephant!

"The labor-delivery rooms are deliberately cosy," Nancy explained. "There are magazines, colored sheets, flowers and an armchair for the father — and women wear their own nightgowns. During delivery the bed is tilted to a 45° angle. Stirrups and draping are not used and there are no spotlights. Only about two in thirty women need episiotomy."

I was particularly interested in the treatment of the newborn in Holland. I'd read Frederick Leboyer's *Birth Without Violence* in which he respects the newborn as a human being, eliminating bright lights, harsh sounds, unduly rough handling and instant clamping and cutting of the cord. It seems that Holland has incorporated these principles for a very long time without any fuss. The births I watched were without spotlights, performed in normal room light. Instructions were minimal and in some cases whispered. The time lapse before cutting the cord varied from two to four minutes. I watched as each baby was placed on its side between the mother's legs and gently massaged. "At the CIZ," Nancy told me, "We also place the baby in a warm bath for a few moments, then it is dressed, nursed and kept at the mother's side."

I believe that this non-violent treatment of the newborn stems from the natural, gentle approach which characterizes the Dutch way of birth. In Holland the mother may choose home birth, safely attended by a nurse-midwife, or give birth in hospital, leaving after 24 hours and visited daily by a doctor for two weeks, or she may stay five to seven days. Babies are examined at the mother's bedside. As Nancy says, "It's all very relaxed and homey."

Amsterdam, population one million, has eight major maternity units, which range from very large to the tiny unit at the CIZ. Procedures vary only slightly across the city. I spoke to a young couple soon expecting their first child. Neliek, a midwife herself, told me they were planning to have the baby in hospital. "If we were in the country we would have our child at home, but since we're in town we feel we might as well go to hospital, as it is just as good. Besides," she added with a laugh, "we live in a tiny apartment several flights of stairs up and the canal below is very busy. We're in the market section of town and there are always trucks around — if we did run into problems an emergency unit would have difficulty getting to me!"

The French Way of Birth

When David and I arrived in France we had high expectations: this is the home of the late Dr. Lamaze, proponent of "psychoprophylaxis"; his equally famous colleague Dr. Pierre Vellay; and most recently, advocate for non-violent birth method, Dr. Frederick Leboyer.

We were able to spend several days at the Château Belvedere, the hospital made famous by Marjorie Karmel in her book, *Thank You Dr. Lamaze.* Shown around by Dr. Vellay, we were impressed by the approach to birth in France, similar to Holland's. The Belvedere is an imposing and gracious building on the outskirts of Paris — the atmosphere calm and friendly. Women in early labor may stroll in the garden and may move freely, eating and drinking lightly. Combination labor-delivery rooms are used, fathers are routinely included and a minimum of interference allows the woman to follow the natural rhythms of labor.

Outstanding at the Belvedere is the "monitrice" or labor coach system, essential to the successful functioning of the childbirth method of "psychoprophylaxis." Women attend classes given by nurses, nurse-midwives or physiotherapists and are coached in muscular control and breathing techniques throughout, often by the same person. At the Belvedere, there are seventeen monitrices. We watched one couple arrive, to be met in the entrance hall by their monitrice, who followed them right through the birth experience. There is no break of "shifts" — the monitrice remains until the child is born, supplementing the emotional support of the father and giving continuity and additional coaching. Routine fetal monitoring is reserved for high risk cases as in Holland — low risk women have their baby's heart-rate checked frequently by a nurse with the standard fetal stethoscope. Dr. Vellay told us, "I do not use routine fetal monitoring, but if it is indicated I will carefully explain to the parents why it is needed." Medication is necessary in fewer than 5% of births here, and as in Holland, verbal sedation is deemed safer and more effective.

I was particularly impressed as I attended the birth of an unprepared Greek woman, a newcomer to France who had had only two sessions to prepare for birth. Throughout the labor, the monitrice used the "watch me-do as I do" coaching technique and the woman remained calm and comfortable. At the time of birth her legs were placed in the French modified stirrups. Her husband, the monitrice and Dr. Vellay encouraged her to a degree I'd rarely seen, and even though the birth required forceps, the woman remained calm through it all. She gave birth with very little pain and required no medication. Impressed, I couldn't help comparing this situation to a similarly unprepared labor in North America — where, too often, even heavy analgesia and anesthesia do not relieve suffering.

Mothers at the Belvedere get up after birth and walk back to their rooms; babies are not separated but stay beside their mothers in a crib. Babies are even examined in their mother's rooms: when David and I were shown the nursery we both exclaimed because it was empty — and remained so in the days we were there. Dr. Vellay proudly showed us the most recent piece of equipment — the latest in infant resuscitators. But he was far prouder of the fact that it had only been needed once in 1974!

The Road to Utopia

In the past five years there have been an astonishing number of changes in methods of childbirth in North America. Many of them have been advocated by books such as this one which stress alternatives in childbirth. The ideas put forward include suggestions that the European experience is one to emulate; that there should be an increase in the use of midwives; that home birth should be more widely practiced; that special maternity centres should be set up; and that existing facilities be refashioned on a more human scale.

Books make suggestions and lay the groundwork, but changes are brought about by people working at the community level for ideas in which they believe. Grassroots childbirth movements have in the past few years organized hundreds of seminars, meetings and conventions; published newsletters; distributed pamphlets and brochures; petitioned hospitals and government in an effort to obtain the kind of childbirth choices they believe best for their area. I'm tremendously heartened by this positive activity, by this outpouring of interest and by the changes it has brought about. Certainly this kind of dedication and enthusiasm is entirely necessary if traditionally North American birth methods are to be changed, for while this kind of activity has been going on, there has been equal activity on the part of those who advocate more, not less, management of birth, a topic I cover in some detail in Chapter Three.

At present, though we may be on the road to Utopia in childbirth, we are still a long way from that goal. At this stage it is still relatively common (though less common all the time) for the advocates of one particular alternative method to believe that theirs is the only possible alternate to the managed birth. The danger of this position is clear. While those groups who favour less intervention in childbirth argue among themselves, the Caesarean rate across the country soars. Home birth, maternity centers, increased use of midwives, birth rooms in hospital, all have excellent points in each of their favours. The important thing for you, in your community, is to work toward getting alternatives in place.

Provided mother, father and baby emerge from the childbirth experience in optimum physical and emotional health with a feeling of achievement, there's no such thing as failure in childbirth. Couples can feel they've failed, however, if their expectations of childbirth can simply not be met in the community. This was brought home forcefully to me several years ago when I received a call from a woman who had recently moved to Montreal and who honestly believed that home birth was the only way to have children. The very idea of doctors and hospitals frightened the daylights out of her. She was equally convinced that classes in prepared childbirth were worse than useless. Yet, at that time in Montreal, the only alternative to a traditional managed birth — other than going it alone — was to find a sympathetic doctor, attend classes and have the child in hospital. She sensed this was true and was on the edge of despair.

Fortunately, I managed to convince her to come to the first couple of classes to see if she thought they might be helpful. She learned relaxation and breathing exercises — and used these tools during labor with her husband lovingly coaching her. Most important she learned communication tools to get the birth of her choice.

Her doctor took her requests seriously. No equipment was used; the birth took place in the labor room; lighting was subdued; no stirrups were used; and the woman gave birth in the position in which she felt most comfortable. The father bathed the baby in warm water right after the birth — he was given permission to bring in a plastic tub in which to do so. A friend who trained in England as a midwife also attended the birth. I'm glad this couple stuck with the classes, and I think they are too.

When I wrote the first edition of this book, I was troubled by the number of parents like the couple previously mentioned. These were bright, concerned people, searching for home birth because they believed that a simple, healthy, dignified birth was unavailable in hospital. Many of these couples felt helpless in the existing obstetrical system. As one woman said, "If I can't get what I want in hospital, I'll have my baby at home." For these parents, the home birth decision was not so much a choice as a cry for help.

One evening a man phoned to tell me that he and his partner were considering a home birth. They had visited a doctor in early pregnancy, but when he told them he wouldn't attend home births, they never went back. They knew nothing of childbirth preparation classes, were living in a semi-rural area about 45 minutes from the city, and the baby was due the next week. The father planned to assist and he was phoning to see if I knew a midwife who might attend. I gave them the name of a general practitioner who had attended home birth, and later asked this doctor about the birth. Their single visit had allowed him to diagnose a feet first position. A healthy baby was born by Caesarean section in a city hospital, the placenta was blocking the cervix — the home birth never attempted.

This is an extreme case. The majority of births are normal; in a country such as Holland, which provides complete preparation, careful screening, midwifery services and back-up, the majority of women can safely choose a home birth. Across North America in recent years, home birth groups have formed, to work to provide the necessary services to make home birth a positive choice, not simply a cry for help.

Since the first edition of this book was published, I have spent many hours discussing the home birth question with parents and professionals. On one occasion, I attended a session for lay-midwives. Ina May Gaskin, author of the book, *Spiritual Midwifery,* talked of the services she and other midwives provided for a rural community in Tennessee. As we watched videotapes of births in that community, I was moved by the obvious love and caring of the midwives. The lay midwives attending the session were operating in a big city where any training or recognition was denied them, and where they were providing birthing attendance, free, to women who refused to go to hospital.

In St. John's, Newfoundland, I spent some time with Hope

Toumishey, director of a new program to train nurse-midwives, in the Nursing Department at Memorial University. She stresses that nurse-midwifery provides continuity of care for the family, not only during pregnancy but through the months of early parenting as well. She complained that although the nurse-midwives are well trained to attend births (deliver babies) at the outpost nursing stations in Newfoundland and Labrador, many women are required to fly to major centers to have their babies delivered by an obstetrician. "Our current obstetrical system is reluctant to accept the role of the nurse-midwife," she told me.

And in Vancouver, B.C., the Campaign Association for the Legalization of Midwifery (CALM) organized, with the Maternal Health Society, a conference entitled, "Midwifery is. . .a labor of love." I firmly believe that this decade will see the training and provision for nurse-midwives to meet an urgent need for the continuity of care which the midwife has traditionally provided — both at home, and in European hospitals.

Home birth has many positive features. The father is able to participate freely, uninhibited by rules. Other children may take part; and the mother can follow her own body rhythms without interference. There is no mother-baby separation, and baby-parent bonding can occur without interruption. But home birth is not for everyone. Even in countries such as Holland and Britain where home birth is made a safe alternative by "flying squads" and superbly trained midwives, many women birth in hospital — and complications can occur no matter how healthy and well-prepared the woman. I was surprised when a British midwife, who had worked in England for fifteen years, told me that she preferred hospital birth to birth at home. "In fifteen years, I only lost one baby — but that's the baby I remember, because it could have been saved if we'd been in a hospital."

Yet home birth provides a warmth and caring that is difficult to duplicate. To witness a woman birthing at home, at one with her body, surrounded by loving family and friends, is an awe-inspiring experience. I've been privileged to share in such events. But without adequate information and support, home birth can be a risky business. Holland's birth system is so "normal" because the majority of women are prepared for birth — and because the back-up system is excellent.

At present, few North American communities offer this kind of support for home birth. However, the hospital "birth room" — a cosy, homey, labor-delivery room — is beginning to appear in some areas, usually as a result of pressure by parents. I believe that the birth room can provide the prepared couple with the best elements of the home birth and hospital birth. Ideally, the birth room offers a friendly, pleasant and supportive atmosphere for labor, delivery, and for parent-child bonding after the baby is born. It also offers parents the security of knowing that, should there be complications, staff and technology will be quickly available. (This new trend will be discussed in detail in Chapter 12).

But what if — like most parts of North America — your community offers neither back-up for home birth, a maternity center, nor a hospital birth room? Don't let this situation depress you. There's every likelihood that if you work within the system, you can have the kind of childbirth you want.

Ultra-Prepared Childbirth

Prepared Childbirth is a safe, acceptable and quite possibly painless alternative to both the passive, medicated "managed" birth and the often uneasy home birth. By "prepared" I differentiate from "natural" as used by those who feel that no preparation is necessary. Prepared Childbirth, correctly taught, is an extremely sophisticated technique, requiring an intimate knowledge of the physiology of childbirth on the part of both the woman and her coach. I doubt that the average twentieth century woman is able to become "one with her body" without preparation. However, almost every woman can experience childbirth as a normal but extremely strenuous activity similar to an athletic event, which in the same way requires dedicated preparation.

Moreover, PC does not exclude the high-risk woman, who also has a right to a fulfilling birth experience.

But unfortunately, the prepared couple is still the exception on this continent, and our obstetrical patterns have become geared to the needs of the majority. Most North American mothers-to-be are unprepared for birth, and gladly accept childbirth drugs and any other "help" the obstetrical staff can offer. In countries where birth is simple and uncomplicated by obstetrical interference — and this includes most of Western Europe — the majority of women are prepared with knowledge, physical fitness and some sort of relaxation and breathing control. Our birthing system will continue to be overly mechanized until every woman is made aware of the need for preparation.

So where does this leave you, the woman expecting a baby? If this is your first baby, you are probably nervous, or at the very least, apprehensive — and quite possibly terrified — of childbirth. If you have already had a child in a typical managed birth, you'll possibly view birth as something to be endured for the sake of the result — your baby. You may have tried some form of Prepared Childbirth and found that it didn't help much, once you got into the hospital.

And what if you're the much-neglected pregnant father? If your mate has had a baby before, you may have been exiled to a waiting room where you imagined untold horrors in the company of other anxious men. Or possibly you were "permitted" in the delivery room, but you didn't really feel you were much help. Or, perhaps this is your first child, and you've never given childbirth much thought. The idea of having a baby appeals to you, but the idea of participating in the birth itself makes you slightly nervous. Or possibly you're looking forward to sharing the pregnancy and participating in the birth as much as possible.

If you're in any of these situations, PC can be the first step to a better birth. But no matter how well you have prepared for the birth itself — with exercises, breathing techniques and mental concentration — hospital policies designed for the unprepared woman may well undermine your efforts. So as well as learning the Lamaze Method or any of its variants, the truly prepared couple will also learn to deal effectively with the obstetrical situation in your hospital.

During the past few years, I've noticed that a large part of my class time is taken up with information about how to work with obstetricians and hospital staff. I've tried to prepare my couples not only for the physical part of childbirth, but to give them psychological preparation so that they can be assertive in the alien, and potentially frightening, world of the doctor and the hospital. Over the years, I've developed some techniques for getting what you want from the obstetrical profession. "Ultra-Prepared Childbirth," (UPC), one of my clients christened my approach, and that's what I call it, for want of a better name.

Thousands of women and men from my classes have put these principles into effect and can testify that, most of the time, they work. Many hospitals across this continent have changed their policies as a result of the communication techniques outlined in this book. I have been tremendously excited by the accounts of parents who have used this book to have the childbirth of their choice.

Dreaming of an obstetrical Utopia, lamenting that it doesn't exist, rejecting the entire system or "putting up" with outmoded birth management routines won't get you an easier, healthier hospital birth. But the UPC techniques I outline in this book should get you most, if not all, of what you want. In the following chapter, you'll see how one couple from my classes successfully used UPC within a fairly typical city hospital.

2 Labor: can you learn to like it?

Jenny and Mario recently shared the birth of their son Tony at a large city hospital. Jenny, 27, is a part time advertising copywriter. Mario, 30, is a full time accountant. Both insist that the only way they can now imagine having a baby is fully prepared.

They attended classes in the psychoprophylactic method of childbirth preparation, practiced each evening together and spent hours discussing birth and choices with other couples and also with their doctor. When labor finally started, both felt confident and excited.

Jenny:

At 2:30 a.m. I woke up with what felt like a menstrual cramp. It was only mild — but it was somehow different from the "Braxton-Hicks" contractions which I'd had before (prelabor contractions). I had ignored these as I knew they were perfectly normal. We'd been told in class, "There's an easy way to decide if it's real labor or not — everything can be taken as false labor until you can no longer ignore it!"

I remembered that my sister — who had scoffed at PC — had leaped out of bed and dragged poor Ed to the hospital at the first cramp — so that both of them were exhausted after at least eight unnecessary hours in the hospital. So I just rolled over on my side and practiced a bit of slow deep breathing, relaxing totally.

I dozed off and woke up again at 5 a.m. with a stronger contraction which I couldn't ignore. "When you can't ignore your contractions just by normal activities it's time to start your slow deep breathing," I remembered. I felt a little guilty about waking Mario but I was so excited I had to.

Mario:

I was surprised at how calm I felt. "Let's time a contraction," I suggested to Jenny, "and see if you can put off using your breathing a bit longer." The contraction was around 50 seconds long — they were about five or six minutes apart — plenty long enough for deep breathing. Using the techniques we'd learned, Jenny relaxed completely and concentrated on breathing during the contraction. In practice sessions, I had always squeezed Jenny's leg hard to "mock" a contraction while she breathed. This had helped her get used to working with a similar sensation to the ones she had started. I massaged her shoulders to help her relax. I timed her contractions, "fifteen seconds . . . thirty seconds (now it's going to ease off) . . . forty five seconds. . ."

Jenny:

As we'd learned to expect, the hardest part of the contraction was about half way through, so when Mario called out "thirty" I knew it was going to get easier. We'd practised this so many times it was second nature. Even though we'd been told that our responses were being conditioned by constant repetition, I had a private fear that maybe I'd forget when it came to the crunch. I was amazed at how automatically I breathed with each contraction.

Mario:

In between contractions, Jenny ate some Jello (traditional Lamaze fare because of its easy digestibility and readily available energy) and emptied her bladder. I called the doctor's answering service and left details of the contractions. I also checked our special bright yellow "Lamaze Goody-Bag" with its load of lollipops, rolling pin, talcum powder, washcloths, Chap-Stick and Jenny's rainbow-striped socks with the toes in them. I also threw in a couple of ham-and-cheese sandwiches and an apple, because I'd been warned that coaching is hard work.

By this time it was 6:30 and the contractions were lasting a good fifty seconds and coming about five minutes apart. Jenny was needing her breathing for each one, but she found that she was most comfortable moving around normally. The night before, she had lost a little of the mucous plug (the protective plug blocking the entrance to the uterus) and now more was coming away. A lot of couples dash to the hospital at the first sign of "bloody show" but we'd been told that this could occur as long as a week before contractions began.

Jenny:

Mario and I had toured the maternity wing of the hospital the week before, so I wasn't at all nervous when I checked in. We had been warned that under this particular hospital's policy, I would be escorted to the labor room in a wheelchair. I was more amused than upset by this welcome, but I certainly could have made it on my own two feet. Anyhow, it gave me a chance to practice my breathing.

Mario:

In class, we had talked about being together for admission and prepping — and one woman, having her second baby, said that she had found that part of the labor the hardest. We asked our doctor, and he told me, "I don't see why you'd want to be there all the time, but it's OK with me — you'll have to check with the nurses, though."

So I walked along with Jenny to the labor area and when the nurses asked me to step into the father's room I told her politely that we had our doctor's permission to be together during admission and examinations. I added that I knew it was far from routine and if it really upset them . . . She told me cheerfully that most men didn't stay for prepping, but if I really wanted to, sure.

Jenny:

I didn't mind the "mini-shave" and the nurse did it quickly, but I had had a really big bowel movement before we left home and I told the nurse that I didn't think I needed one and that I was nervous of enemas. I had discussed that earlier with my doctor, too, and he'd said that maybe I could avoid it. I could see the nurse wondering if we were going to give her trouble, so I told her that Mario and I really appreciated being together. She didn't say another word about the enema — I think she was too busy to argue.

Just then, an intern walked in with a sheaf of papers and told me he'd like to ask me a few questions. I explained that I was using the Lamaze method of prepared childbirth and wouldn't talk when I was having a contraction. He seemed surprisingly ignorant about it, but said, "Sure." I was really pleased that Mario was with me, because he knew the answers to most of the questions.

After that, a resident came in to examine me internally and I was really thankful for Mario. The resident asked him to step outside for a moment but Mario told her, "We've got Dr. B's permission to be together." The resident looked a bit surprised, and I thought she might insist that Mario leave, but she simply shrugged and both of us heaved a sigh of relief.

Mario:

Jenny found it quite hard to relax during the internal, so I asked her to look straight at me and change to her light, more rapid breathing which seemed to give her more control. When it was over, she asked how far dilated her cervix was, and the doctor said four centimeters. We knew that the longest part of labor is getting up to 4 cm, so we were pretty pleased with ourselves.

Jenny:

I had a fetal monitor strapped on. I'd been warned about this but I still felt a bit claustrophobic and a little inhibited. I had asked beforehand if my baby's heart could be monitored simply by the nurse. The doctor told me that if I was lucky, all four of the hospital's monitors would be in use, and I wouldn't have to be attached to one. As it turned out though, there was one available. The doctor had told us that the hospital had to use all available equipment — or risk malpractice suits — so I was stuck with it. Mario tried to settle me into some comfortable position. I wound up sitting tailor fashion with the head of the bed rolled up as far as possible.

Mario:

I was really busy at this point. During contractions, I coached Jenny and between them I would fill in the labor log that I was keeping. Our instructor had suggested that this would be helpful to give us an idea of labor progress, and what to do when. Fortunately, Jenny wasn't having any backache, so the rolling pin stayed in the yellow bag.

Jenny:

The nurse who had prepped me didn't seem to know much about the breathing, but she didn't try to interfere with it. But then her shift finished and we really had a good break. A young nurse came in and said, "Hi, I hear you're using the Lamaze Method. It's fantastic! I've seen quite a few couples using it and it really works. Just let me know if there's anything I can do to help."

Mario:

We really felt good, just knowing that somebody was with us. It was a hot July day, and the labor room wasn't air-

conditioned. Simply by bringing some chipped ice for Jenny to suck on, without our asking, she really boosted our morale.

We found that most of the staff were pleasant, although not awfully familiar with what we were doing — except for one incident. Our hospital is a teaching hospital and we had asked the nurse not to let students come in during our labor because we didn't want to break Jenny's concentration. But at one point a young man — a total stranger! — in street clothing and no name tag, asked me to step outside and said to Jenny, "Okay, spread your legs."

Jenny:

Mario looked furious, but before I could say anything, he calmly told the man, "I don't think we know who you are, and my wife has just been examined."

Mario:

He seemed surprised that anyone would question him — but he turned and left without a word. Later, the nurse told us he was an intern, and nobody knew why he was there!

Jenny:

By this time it was 10 a.m. My contractions had been lasting a minute or so and coming every three minutes for the last hour or so. I was in a pattern of accelerating my breathing as soon as a contraction began and easing it right off by about twenty seconds. Mario was great.

Mario:

Then suddenly Jenny had this huge contraction. I could see her tense up, and for a moment I thought she was losing control. I remembered the instructor saying that this might happen and it was really important for me to get her back on the track. I said to Jenny, "Look at me. Relax your shoulders. Breathe with me."

And almost instinctively we moved into the light rhythmic

breathing which we had practiced to the tune of Yankee Doodle. When the contraction stopped, Jenny said, "Whew, that was a biggie! I don't think I can take too many more of those. I'm starting to have backache."

We'd learned that the prepared woman might move quickly once her cervix hit four centimeters but I didn't think she'd move this quickly. I rolled the bed down, and got Jenny lying on her side. I sprinkled some talcum powder on her back and for the next contraction massaged her back the way we had practiced. Jenny really needed her Yankee Doodle breathing. If I hadn't been keeping my review sheet, I would have thought she was using it too soon. But the contractions were lasting ninety seconds and coming only a minute apart. Jenny was getting restless, and I could see her confidence begin to waver.

Jenny:

I guess the lowest part of the labor came right then. Our nice nurse had gone to lunch, and another nurse walked in. Mario said to her, "I think my wife is coming into transition."*

"I really don't think she can be in transition," the nurse told him. "She was only four centimeters a little while ago. She's got about another five hours to go so she'd better slow down her breathing. I'll see about getting an epidural organized."

Mario:

We'd gone over medication and anesthetics in detail in the PC classes, and while we both agreed that if it were really

---

* *There is a period of about an hour preceding the actual birth, sometimes called the "hurricane hour" or the "transition period", in which the contractions become hard and erratic, very close together, and may be accompanied by a number of symptoms such as hiccups, leg shaking, nausea, extreme irritability, back pain, and eventually an urge to push. At this time, the unprepared woman will normally lose all control.*

necessary, Jenny would decide to have an epidural, we felt that we were well enough equipped with our techniques for an epidural to be unnecessary unless there was a complication.

Jenny:
Initially I wasn't one of those women who really wanted to go through birth without medication, but I'd had a few friends who'd had epidurals that they weren't delighted with, and I had done a little bit of reading about possible effects of any medication on the baby. So I decided that if I were in control with my techniques, I'd like to try not to have anything. In a way, I guess, I also wanted to feel what it was like to give birth without having my sensation cut off.

But when the nurse said five hours, *I panicked. "I can't go on," I told Mario. The nurse was waiting outside. "I want an epidural," I said.*

Mario:
Poor Jenny was almost in tears. I was positive *this was transition. Our instructor had told us that often the prepared woman will move faster through labor than hospital staff is used to, and this seemed to be the situation with Jenny. I stroked her hand. "Do you think you can hang on through twenty contractions like this? They're not going to get any worse, and I'm sure we're going to have our baby in an hour or so."*

Jenny sniffled and said, "Yeah, I guess so. As long as they don't get any worse." The nurse popped her head back inside the door and asked if Jenny had decided to have an epidural. I told her we'd like to wait for a while. She wasn't unpleasant, and said, "Just call me if you need me . . .Don't feel bad about having an epidural. Most women do."

Then a funny thing happened. Jenny's legs started to shake. Aha, I thought. It's certainly *transition! I said to Jenny, "Hey, that's great. Your legs are shaking."*

Jenny snapped back, "Yeah, what's great about that? Could you stop breathing all over me? All this hot air is bothering me. "

For a moment I felt hurt. Then I realized that this was a variation of the don't-touch-me set of responses normal for transition. So I kept rubbing Jenny's back and we Yankee Doodled some more.

Jenny:

About sixteen contractions had gone by and suddenly I got a really weird sensation — almost as though I had to have a bowel movement. I grunted to Mario, "I've gotta push."

Mario snapped, "Blow . . . blow . . . blow . . ." and rang the bell for the nurse. She came and stuck her head around the door. "Jenny feels like pushing . . . could we have her examined?" he asked.

Mario:

*She looked a bit cynical but went away and came back with the woman resident who had examined Jenny before. "Oh, my God," she said. For one awful moment, I was afraid there was something wrong. Then I remembered being told about the "Oh, my God Syndrome" which means that the baby is coming earlier than they anticipated. * Then things really started moving.*

Our nice nurse was just back from lunch, and she showed me where to change for the delivery. I made it to the delivery room just as Jenny was wheeled in. "Blow, Jenny," I instructed her.

I helped the nurse lift Jenny onto the delivery table, and reminded her that Jenny had her doctor's permission not to use stirrups. "Fine," said the nurse.

"Where's the doctor?" asked Jenny, suddenly wide-awake and full of energy. "Feel like delivering the baby, Mario?"

---

* The cervix of the prepared woman dilates more rapidly from 4 to 10 cm, because she is relaxed. But most hospital staff regard the longer dilation time — and slower labor — of the unprepared woman as the norm, hence the "Oh, my God!"

Our doctor's colleague entered the room. I thought there might be some problem over the stirrup thing, but he didn't insist. I took my place at Jenny's head and the doctor gave her the okay to go ahead and push. Because lying on your back is not the most comfortable position to deliver a child in, I asked our nurse for more pillows, and she managed to find two more. While Jenny pushed, I supported her head, shoulders and three pillows to lift her into a comfortable, almost semi-sitting position while she supported her legs flat on her chest and apart.

Jenny:

I was really surprised that I knew exactly how to push. Somebody — I don't know who it was — told me to push into my bottom as though I were having a large bowel movement. But in the back of my mind I remembered being told in class that this kind of pushing would increase my chance of hemorrhoids. So I tried to relax my rectum and push into the vagina as I had learned . . . "Down . . . up . . . and out . . ." It felt so good to push. Somebody asked me if I wanted the mirror, but all I wanted was to close my eyes and push my child down . . . up . . . and out.

In my ear, I could her Mario's voice counting while I held my breath. "One. . .two. . .three. . .thirteen, fourteen, fifteen. . .release." I let just enough breath out to stop from exploding, inhaled deeply and pushed.

Suddenly I felt a slight burning sensation at the vaginal outlet. I knew the head must be crowning. I had discussed with my doctor whether it would be possible not to have an episiotomy if it wasn't really necessary. I didn't think of it at the time, and I guess I was really lucky because my doctor's colleague said to me, "I think you may be able to get by without an episiotomy, just lie back and pant."

I did. I could feel the baby's head being eased out. Then my doctor asked me to give one more push for the shoulders and for a split second I felt as though I were being torn apart. And then the baby was out, and it was fantastic! It was crying im-

mediately, and Mario was hugging me and we were so excited we forgot to ask what it was.

"It's a boy," said the doctor. He placed him on my tummy and he was a beautiful pink, and after his first healthy scream or two, seemed perfectly calm. It was so beautiful . . . we were both crying.

Mario:
I don't think I have ever been so moved. It was just incredible. This beautiful little pink baby coming out and me holding Jenny up to look at our child. I really felt we had done it together. I forget exactly what happened then. I think the placenta came away, and because Jenny didn't need any stitches, the nurse gave me the baby, to hold for a moment, and then I gave him to Jenny. I remember being knocked out by his perfect little fingers and funny long fingernails.

Jenny:
I'd asked to nurse my baby right away, and I'll never forget the feeling when he first started to suckle. I can't imagine doing it any other way. Mario and I felt closer than we'd ever felt before, and even though Tony is nine months now, we still feel really close over him, and we'll never forget his birth.

What Is Prepared Childbirth?

Jenny and Mario are typical of the couples in my classes. They arrived for the first class somewhat nervously — attending only because they were urged to do so by friends who had had a prepared childbirth six months previously.

At the first class, which I schedule as soon as possible in pregnancy, we discuss the couple's expectations and their feelings about birth, cultural attitudes and the historical view of pain in childbirth. We cover a brief history of childbirth education, beginning with Grantly Dick-Read's beliefs that pain in childbirth is the result of fear — fear produced by generations of "old wives' tales" and a negative approach to birth. We discuss Read's "Natural Childbirth" education program to eliminate fear and thus pain by knowledge, physical fitness and relaxation. Then we progress to the Russian method of reducing pain in childbirth, based on the scientific principles of Pavlovian conditioning.

By this method, known as "psychoprophylaxis" (sometimes called PPM), the brain can be taught to select a response to a given stimuli. When labor begins, the brain of the unprepared, fearful woman selects the response "Tense — hold your breath", which leads to Read's "fear-tension-pain" cycle. But the prepared woman using conditioning is trained by constant repetition to select the response "Breathe — release your muscles — work". By a set of precise exercises, the woman learns to control all her voluntary muscles. Even under the stress of actual labor, the prepared woman will be able to raise her pain threshold, conserve energy, and allow the involuntary muscles of the uterus to operate without hindrance from other tense muscles. Breathing techniques vary with the intensity of the contraction and work physiologically with the changing phases of labor. Preparing for labor, she practises muscular control and breathing techniques until they become automatic — in much the same way that an experienced driver learns to shift the gear positions of a standard shift car without thinking. In labor, reinforced by the coach, her brain selects the responses "Breathe — release muscles" to the stimulus of a contraction.

We discuss the idea of "painless childbirth", what each woman can expect realistically, and the role of medication in obstetrics, when necessary. About one-third of the women from my classes will later describe labor as totally painless; the other two-thirds will freely admit to some physical pain made totally bearable by the techniques. My own childbirth experience was of some physical pain — had I stopped to analyze it — which I would compare to the pain I recall as a high school hurdler bursting through the finish line. Like an athlete, the face of even a prepared woman in childbirth is often contorted, as if in great pain — but her mind is so centered on achieving her goal that the pain becomes secondary, and is in many cases unnoticed. I can't guarantee that the prepared woman will have a totally painless childbirth. But what I can guarantee to almost all prepared women is childbirth without *suffering.* By suffering, I mean passively — and possibly even stoically — enduring pain with which one is not prepared to cope.

Because the prepared woman approaches childbirth relaxed, knowledgeable and equipped to work *with* (not against) contractions, she will probably not require medication or anesthetic. More than 80% of the women in my classes find that they do not need drugs of any kind. However, the prepared woman also understands that in the event of complication — such as Caesarean birth, for example — anesthesia and other high-risk procedures may be necessary. In such cases, "preparation" means being able to co-operate fully with the medical staff. The prepared woman knows that her baby's safety — and her own — are far more important than the exact method of birth. (Many doctors and nurses have remarked on the ability of the prepared couple to work calmly throughout even the most complicated labor.)

A large part of the class is spent discussing the role of the father as labor "coach" and the benefits to man and woman from a shared childbirth. The class finishes with an outline of the anatomy and physiology of pregnancy and labor; physical side-effects of pregnancy; how to minimize any discomfort by excellent posture; and the importance of physical fitness, superior nutrition and an ultra-conservative approach to drugs in pregnancy. (See Chapter 6.) We conclude by discussing emotional attitudes and changes of both men and women during pregnancy. By the end of the class, usually the initial apprenhension has dissolved, and I can sense more than a flickering of interest in even those men who were reluctant to attend.

This class is followed by a session on nutrition in pregnancy and its importance, then by a class of exercises designed to firm muscles under stress in pregnancy for maximum comfort and a rapid return to normal after birth, together with introduction to the facts of breastfeeding.

Eight weeks before the birth — usually enthusiastic and highly motivated by this time — couples return for intensive learning of the practice of the Russian method (psychoprophylaxis) often called by the name of its French variation, "Lamaze Method".

At weekly classes which continue until the birth, couples begin the basis of muscular control — the ability to tense or relax any group of voluntary muscles at will. Women start by tensing an arm or leg, keeping everything else totally relaxed. Right away, the coach notices that his partner is holding her breath and everything else has tensed as well — a good illustration of what happens to the unprepared woman during a contraction! Assisted by her coach, the woman breaks this pattern by concentrating on relaxing everything but the working muscles and breathing slowly and normally. As the coach gives instructions he quickly becomes expert at locating tension, helping his partner relax by massage and verbal cues. His partner progresses to tensing (contracting) several body parts — then after a week of practice, learns to tense many parts of her body. Finally, by the end of the course she will be able to contract many small muscle groups, keeping everything else totally relaxed. This is the sort of control she'll need in the labor situation when the involuntary muscles of the uterus are contracting. By this time, she'll be able to remain relaxed with the help of her coach, even in a busy labor unit while she's having very strong contractions — no easy feat!

Next come the breathing techniques, used in labor much like the gears of a car. There are three stages of labor. A longish first stage to thin out (efface) and dilate the opening of the uterus (cervix) to ten centimeters, then a shorter, very vigorous second stage, during which the mother will push her baby out, then a brief third stage to expel the placenta.

For a good part of the first stage, contractions can be easily ignored. When she can no longer ignore them by normal activities, the woman uses a slow, deep, chest breathing to work with each contraction. When this breathing ceases to "work" with stronger contractions, she switches to a shallower breathing higher in the chest — progressing to controlled, light mouth breathing at the "peak" of the contraction. A light rhythmic mouth breathing, with regular emphasis on the breath out to a rhythm such as "Yankee Doodle" (kept by the coach), is used when the previous breathing is no longer effective. A blowing technique is taught to control a premature "urge to push" and correct breathing and muscular control are learned for the expulsion of the baby.

Because I believe that a couple must be prepared for the *most difficult labor possible,* we spend considerable time on variations from the norm. I teach a technique which conditions both the man and woman to regain control, should this waver under the stress of intense contractions, which is quite common.

The conditioned response is developed by consistent verbal cues, given by the coach — "Contraction begins" — at which his partner responds immediately with muscular release, a breathing pattern, a light abdominal massage called *effleurage* and concentration on some small object such as a photograph ("focal point"). After daily practice, her responses to his cues become automatic. After several weeks Mario and Jenny assured the class that conditioning had occurred. "I decided to test it out on Jenny at supper," Mario explained. "In the middle of the meal I snapped, "Contraction begins" and Jenny responded just the way we'd been practicing. Then we knew her responses were automatic!"

Because it is important to learn to work with a real sensation, I have the coach always apply pressure to the thigh or upper leg, grading the pressure to produce a change in breathing techniques. Couples report that by the end of the course it's difficult to stimulate any pain threshold at all by simply "pinching" — the pain threshold has gradually become higher. "It was so much easier in labor," quipped

Mario, "I didn't have to pinch!"

We watch films of birth and baby care, discuss with other parents their experiences, go through hospital procedures in detail, review the high-risk labor and spend rather a large part of the course discussing "how to get what you want by working with the staff . . ."

Jenny and Mario had a near-perfect "un-natural" (but non-medicated) childbirth — but only because of their own efforts. Not only were they prepared physically and mentally for the actual birth, they were "Ultra-Prepared" to deal with the hospital situation. They had checked out all aspects of the birth with the doctor — well in advance — and during labor and delivery they used firmness and conviction in dealing with well-meaning medical staff who offered them a more "mechanized" delivery. The birth would have been *absolutely* perfect, Jenny and Mario say, if the fetal monitor had not been used, if Jenny could have given birth in the labor rooms, and if everyone on the staff had been familiar with the Lamaze Method and realized that a prepared woman generally has a faster labor.

By the time childbirth is imminent, each couple should function as a team, in much the same way as Jenny and Mario did. And a good childbirth class should equip each couple to continue to act as an assertive team, after their baby is born. For example, following the birth, my own course includes a section on "Parenting", which will be discussed in more detail in Chapter 7.

Can you learn to like labor? Maybe *like* is too strong a word, but certainly a woman can learn to respond positively to the sensations of childbirth — so that both partners will recall the event as a joyful and loving experience. Unfortunately, today in North America, only a handful of hospitals give total support to Prepared Childbirth. Even many of our so-called "enlightened" hospitals routinely impede the progress of normal labor by insisting on outmoded routines. In the following chapter, we'll take a hard look at the routines the prepared parent may wish to avoid.

3   What price the managed birth?

When we got to the hospital on D-Day, the hospital staff was determined to steer me in the general direction of the men's washroom, almost assuredly not in the direction of the labor room. First they separate you from your wife when the little old lady at the desk hits you with some forms to fill out; name, rank, serial number, all that.

"Look," I said, "I'm in the middle of something kinda important; can those wait 'til later?" I started hotfooting it towards the stairwell.

Up three flights of stairs and I ask a custodian where the labor rooms are, and he says, "There . . . but YOU can't go in."

One step to the door of the labor room now and this intern pipes, "You can't come in here."

By now I've heard this tune twice and I tell the guy, "Sure I can come in here . . . MY DOCTOR SAID SO!" Strategic little lie, but not an unwarranted one.

"OK," he says grudgingly. "But stay outta the way."

*Then this other intern walks up with a sheet of things to
fill out. The questions are a riot, 'specially since we're
trying to get a little Lamaze action going: Wife's age
. . . birthplace . . . has she ever had cholera? Has she
ever had bubonic plague? . . . and on and on.*
                                    — *Bill Mann, newspaper reporter.*

Bill Mann's experience is a fairly typical one, although his
creatively stubborn reaction may not be. His wife's labor was
progressing rapidly. She needed his support and he wanted to
provide it. The objection? Hospital routine, or "policy".

Too frequently, normal, low-risk birth is "managed" by a
whole set of obstetrical interferences. Many of these "policies" and routines have been shown conclusively by an ever-
growing body of scientific literature on human birth to be
damaging to both mother and baby. At the very least, they
make the whole experience of childbirth far less comfortable
for all concerned.

Admission And Prepping

Admission forms and medical questionnaires generally
cause needless interruptions for the woman and her coach.
Why can't questionnaires be completed in advance and mailed to the hospital or presented on arrival? If a lengthy
medical questionnaire must be filled out, then why not at least
let the father provide the information, while his partner concentrates on breathing techniques and comfort?

Routine pubic shaves and enemas are of dubious advantage
to the woman. Although the once routine complete pubic
shave has been replaced by a "mini-shave" at most hospitals,
most women would prefer clipping. "I remember the itching
and prickling when the hair was growing back," Andrea F.
says. "That may not sound like much, but when you have to
wear a pad for a couple of weeks and you're sore from
episiotomy it amounts to a lot — if shaving could be avoided
a lot of women would be much more comfortable."

Routine shaving is done chiefly to facilitate episiotomy and its repair and is said to prevent infection. In "The Cultural Warping of Childbirth", Doris Haire cites one study involving 7,600 women. According to Haire, women with no shave had a lower infection rate than those who had been shaved![1]

It is true that an enema can prevent unnecessary discomfort in late labor and may also remove possible fear of having a bowel movement on the delivery table, which might inhibit a woman's pushing. But nature generally goes to work without an enema: most women have the urge to defecate in early labor and for many this takes the form of diarrhea. Needless enemas can cause undue discomfort — and even cause women to lose the control needed for prepared childbirth techniques. "I told the nurse that I'd had diarrhea at home," Karen W. told me, "but she insisted that I have an enema, even though my cervix was almost fully dilated. Up until then I'd been totally in control. She sent my husband out and the enema made the contractions so strong that I lost control — I still feel she was needlessly cruel."

Routine Fetal Heart Monitors

The fetal heart monitor was strapped on too tight and I was very uncomfortable . . . it gave me claustrophobia. I had backache and I kept trying to find a comfortable position and the nurse kept coming in and asking me to lie on my back because I was causing "static."
—Judy F.

They hooked me up to a fetal monitor and I could watch the contractions, and my baby's heartbeat, on the screen. When I lay back, closed my eyes, and practised my breathing, everything was fine. But the minute I stopped concentrating and looked at the screen, even a small contraction became unbearably painful.
— Christiane M.

In 1972 I listened as Elisabeth Bing deplored the trend towards mechanization and consequent depersonalization of childbirth in the United States. Speaking at a conference of the International Childbirth Education Association, she described fetal heart monitors, external and internal, used routinely throughout labor and the common practice of setting up an intravenous drip (IV) on admission. I was pregnant and relieved that these procedures were not routine in Canada, but were reserved for "high-risk" labors only. Women in normal labor were checked regularly by a nurse, who recorded the heart rate with a regular fetal stethoscope.

I escaped the fetal monitor and the IV. But by 1974, most women in large U.S. and Canadian hospitals were "hooked up" to expensive equipment during the entire labor; many women were being given IV's "just in case" exhaustion set in or an emergency cropped up. Before 1974, I had been able to give my couples fairly simple descriptions of hospital procedures for normal labor. But today, my classes seem to have turned into seminars discussing equipment and high-risk procedures. Seminars in which the question, "But why is it necessary?" is increasingly difficult to answer.

There are two methods of monitoring the baby's heartbeat throughout labor. The least complicated is an external attachment strapped to the woman's abdomen, and attached to a loudspeaker for all to hear. The other method is an internal device which requires rupture of the membranes. Electrodes are attached to the skin of the baby's scalp; his/her heart rate is recorded on a graph in a box-like machine by the side of the woman's bed. Many women complain of discomfort during this insertion, particularly if a contraction occurs. In the case of high-risk pregnancy, internal monitoring is chosen because of its greater accuracy: fetal heart distress is picked up immediately and many Caesarean sections have been performed, based on the monitor's findings.

The external monitor is sensitive to vibrations from other bodily functions: sounds and tracings can be disturbed by changes in the mother's position. Thus, some degree of immobility is required: most women are asked to lie on their backs. And this position may actually *trigger* the fetal distress the equipment is designed to detect! When the woman labors on her back, two large blood vessels near her heart are compressed, reducing blood flow and oxygen to the baby — often producing a slowdown in fetal heart rate (FHR).

Dr. Roberto Caldeyro-Barcia, President of the International Federation of Gynecologists and Obstetricians not only relates abnormal FHR to immobility caused by monitoring, but also questions the practice of artificial rupture of amniotic membranes required to install the internal fetal monitor. He has documented that artificial rupture in early labor can damage the baby's skull and brain as well as speed up labor dangerously.[2]

Similarly, physical therapist Madeleine Shearer writes, "Since the high risk fetuses are the most vulnerable to head and cord compression we may wonder whether some of the abnormal heart rates are due to loss of protective fluid occasioned by internal monitoring."[3] (The effects of artificially rupturing the amniotic membranes will be discussed in more detail in following pages.)

And in June 1974, the editor of *Obstetrical and Gynecological Survey* writes, "The incidence of Caesarean section operation is increased when internal monitoring techniques are used."[4]

Shearer also believes that the position used for monitoring possibly contributes to such distress. She notes that because laboratory tests needed to confirm distress are often delayed or not possible, Caesarean section is performed immediately.[5]

McLennan and Sandberg, in their textbook, *Synopsis of Obstetrics*, state the incidence of Caesarean section as 4-6%, adding that "in some institutions the rate for private patients is 9-10% and invariably the rate is higher than that for clinic patients"[6] Staff or clinic patients, — usually underprivileged — are traditionally given less medication, and less equipment throughout labor. In the light of recent findings, poverty may be a blessing in the delivery room. Estimates for Caesarean Section in many large teaching hospitals run as high as 25% and many of these are performed following fetal distress detected by monitoring.

In one report on fetal monitoring in a Manitoba hospital, the authors conclude: "Caesarean sections were at times done for obstetricians' distress instead of fetal distress. Fetal blood sampling was not used to refine decisions." At this hospital, "C-section" rate was 22% for monitored patients, compared to 8.5% for non-monitored patients.[7]

Shearer and other attribute the soaring use of fetal monitors to pressure from monitor companies who may stress dangers of birth and the possibility of lawsuits to obstetricians who do not use the available equipment. "I don't use monitors routinely, I don't approve of it," says one doctor. "But if a hospital has three monitors and doesn't use all, it's open to malpractice suit."

Monitor companies have funded, staffed and equipped research centers in large teaching hospitals. No wonder these centers show that the monitor can reduce perinatal mortality! Although the rate of Caesarean Section has decreased in centers where routine monitoring has been used for years, the rate tends to increase where it has recently been introduced. Possibly as time goes on, the attendants become more skilled at interpreting monitor tracings.

I don't deny that fetal monitoring can be of particular help in high-risk labors. But I also agree with Shearer's suggestion that parents whose babies are monitored have a right to an accurate explanation of the need for such a procedure and an opportunity to give what she refers to as "informed consent".

Intravenous Fluids

I arrived at the hospital on the verge of transition. I was completely in control and had been in labor only a few hours. The nurse insisted that she set up an IV "just in case".

"Just in case what?" I asked.

"Well, you might get exhausted, and if you hemorrhaged it would be easier to manage if you have the IV."

*But I was about to have the baby and I wasn't even
tired! As far as hemorrhaging goes, I'm sure they could
do something pretty quickly if that did happen, but is
that so common? By the time they got that set up, I was
having a hard time controlling the urge to push . . .*
— *Dot B.*

The North American woman entering a large hospital is
likely to have an intravenous attachment set up, connecting a
vein in her arm, by means of a thin tube, to a bottle on a bedside stand. She will be told that this will give her glucose
during the hours when she must not eat and drink, that it
keeps a vein open "Just in case" an emergency occurs and
transfusions are necessary. The IV is promptly set up and the
woman labors with some degree of immobility. If she is using
psychoprophylactic techniques, she is unable to perform the
light abdominal massage (*effleurage*) which she has practised.
She is confined to bed and must use a bedpan instead of a toilet. Staff will pop in frequently and adjust her IV. The IV attachment also provides easy access for administration of
simulated oxytocin (used to produce or stimulate contraction)
to speed the labor process.

One older doctor told me, "It's a newfangled thing. In my
day we didn't feel there was enough risk in normal labor to
justify hooking every woman up to an IV. We left that sort of
thing for when it was really needed. And things didn't go
wrong any more than they do now . . . maybe less."

Doris Haire writes, "The effect on the fetus of depriving
the mother of food and drink for many hours as is the custom
in the United States has not been sufficiently investigated.
Intravenous feeding as a substitute for light eating only adds
to the pathologic environment of the American hospital.

One investigation does point to negative side effects from
intravenous fluids. Doctors Altstatt (1965) and Battaglia,
1960, found that intravenous fluids cause "electrolyte imbal-
ance and lethargy, poor muscle tone and color" in the newborn infant.[9]

Recent work by Dr. Ronald Myers at the National Institute of Neurological and Communicative Disorders, Bethesda, Maryland, indicates a need for caution in giving routine IV's. His studies suggest that when the brain is deprived of oxygen, the resulting damage to the brain is caused by the buildup of lactic acid in the brain. He believes that the extent of lactic accumulation is directly related to the amount of glucose in the blood just before the circulation is stopped. Rhesus monkeys with an IV of glucose suffered most brain damage when circulation was stopped.[9a]

In most countries of the world women are permitted to eat and drink lightly in early labour. Yet when Carol. A. arrived at the hospital and an examination showed her cervix to be a mere centimeter dilated, a nurse proceeded to set up an IV and told her, "You musn't eat or drink in hospital, because if you needed a general anesthetic for a Caesarean section you might vomit and that can be fatal."

Though Caesarean births are on the increase, a steadily increasing number are performed under regional anesthesia, which is quite safe even if the woman has eaten recently. Even if the woman has not eaten throughout labor, the stomach is not completely empty. In view of these facts, routine IV to replace light snacking seems overly cautious and unnecessary.

Routine IV's for normal labor are of questionable benefit to the woman, yet most women are made to believe that without such precautions something terrible will happen. As Doris Haire says, the IV adds to the pathological environment of the obstetrical unit.

Induced Labor

My doctor told me that she'd be out of town the next week — when my baby was due — and that she could "bring me in" a week early.

I went in the night before and they started the IV first thing next morning. I had to have a monitor strapped

*on. The IV and monitor were not painful but I had to keep
fairly still . . . The contractions were mild at first, then
they got really strong all at once and I could hardly cope
with them. People kept fiddling with the drip
and when they examined me my cervix hadn't
progressed at all.*

*They speeded things up and the contractions became
almost unbearable. So they turned the drip down . . .
then everything seemed to stop. For about four hours, I
had terribly strong contractions almost one on top of
another.*

*Finally they gave me an epidural and that helped a
bit, but everything started to slow down again. The
baby needed forceps and she was only six pounds. She
had problems with breastfeeding and wouldn't suck
well. Maybe it was all coincidence but I can't help feeling that she wasn't really ready to be born.*

— Janet M.

Induction is the process of bringing about the onset of labor, either by rupturing the amniotic membranes or by giving
the woman simulated oxytocin, orally or intravenously, either
to produce or to stimulate uterine contractions. Doctors who
induce only for medical reasons estimate that fewer than 5%
of mothers *need* to be induced. As Janet discovered, induction can be a painful process. It can also be dangerous to the
infant, according to the textbook *Synopsis of Obstetrics*,
which states, "Elective induction merely for convenience of
the patient or physician may be associated with various hazards — prematurity, intrapartum infections after a prolonged labor, or prolapse of the cord."[10]

For some time I was not aware of the burst of induced
labors in Montreal. Then, one evening Dr. R. phoned me.
"I'd like you to tell your classes that induction is a routine
thing now. I'm inducing about 85% of my patients about a
week before the due date. It's better for both of us: I don't
work well in the middle of the night and it's easier for the

woman to deliver a smaller baby in a shorter labor. Waiting for the baby to come is old-fashioned. Induction is the wave of the future," he added.

Shocked, I discussed this conversation with an obstetrician friend who rarely induces. "One day he's going to run into trouble . . . he'll get a baby who is just not ready to come," he commented.

Induction for convenience has spread to other countries. One Australian doctor agrees it's a risky business. Speaking at a 1974 conference of obstetricians and gynecologists at Melbourne University, Dr. Noel De Garis cited some shocking figures. In Victoria, Australia, 28 babies died of every 1,000 in which labor had been induced for no other reason than the doctor's convenience — compared to only 17 deaths per 1,000 babies born without induction! De Garis believes that unless there are adequate staff of sufficient experience, expensive electronic equipment and facilities for operating an intensive care unit, the method should be discontinued.[11]

In a large Montreal hospital recently, one baby died in induction circumstances which were far removed from these standards. The mother was one of my clients. Heartbroken, she phoned to talk with me. Induction had been used to accelerate labor, the heartbeat was not monitored and the mother was left alone with contractions which she described as incredibly strong and one on top of another. When the nurse returned after supper break the heart beat had stopped. Perhaps induction did not cause the baby's death — but inadequate management of the procedure could well have played a part.

Dr. Roberto Caldeyro-Barcia believes that in as many as 90% of inductions the procedure is unnecessary. Even when used under ideal conditions, oxytoxic drugs produce contractions which are too strong and may cause a reduction of oxygen to the baby's brain, he states. Caldeyro-Barcia also believes that the common practice of artificially rupturing the amniotic membranes is not in the best interests of either mother or baby. The amniotic fluid protects the head and cord. Premature rupturing — and the loss of this fluid — may cause uneven pressure on the head, with resulting misalignment of the skull bones and marked elongation or "molding". Studies show that where such misalignment occurs, there is possible damage to underlying blood vessels and the brain.

He adds that early rupture of the membranes may cause an increase of pressure during contractions: fetal heart monitors show a marked decrease in oxygen to the baby — a rare occurrence if the membranes are intact. His studies indicate that if the membranes are not ruptured artificially, 95% will rupture in very late labor, just prior to delivery. If they are ruptured at 4-5 cms (the common practice), misalignment of the skull bones occurs more frequently than in late ruptured cases.

It's ironic that artificial rupturing of the membranes seems to speed up labor by only 30-40 minutes. Barcia asks, "Is it worthwhile to reduce labor by 30-40 minutes at the expense of all the deformation and possible damage to the head of the fetus? My feelings are that it is not worthwhile; we should not interfere with the normal process. Nature has organized labor, keeping intact the membranes up to the last phase of labor in the majority of women."[12]

"Overdue" or "On Time"?

Induction has become almost routine for the woman who goes two weeks beyond her given due date. Colorado physician Dr. Robert Bradley, vigorous proponent of non-medicated childbirth, condemns this trend. "If you take all the eight pound babies that had spontaneous labor without induction, you'll find that 80% of them are born two weeks after that stupid "due date". That's because doctors count from the last menstrual period rather than from conception . . . These forced births are premature. We know this practice is responsible in many cases for the high incidence of hyaline membrane disease — many of these babies simply aren't ready for the task of breathing on their own yet."[13]

Among my own clients, 80% of the babies arrive approximately two weeks past the given due date — all of these "late babies" have been healthy and an excellent birth weight.

Drugs and Anesthesia

When I arrived at the hospital, I was feeling fine. I was having contractions that needed only slow deep breathing and I wasn't in pain. The nurse told me that the doctor had ordered a sedative to help me relax . . . "to help me with my exercises." I took the pill and began to feel pleasantly drowsy. But as contractions got harder, I couldn't concentrate on my breathing. By the time my cervix was five cm dilated, I had almost given up trying to concentrate, and I asked for something to help me with the pain I was feeling.

The nurse said it was too early for epidural but I was given a shot of Demerol, to "take the edge off" my contractions. As that wore off, they told me I was ready for my epidural and most women needed one . . .

It seemed to take ages before I was ready to deliver. I didn't feel any urge to push so the doctor used forceps. The worst part was, I started out so well. Although I wasn't opposed to medication, I'm sure that if I hadn't had that sedative I could have handled most of the labor. The attitude was that no one could have a baby without anesthetics, so why bother trying?

— Angela B.

If you're a woman in labor or delivery, you may be administered sedatives, hypnotics, tranquilizers, analgesics or anesthetics, or, more likely a combination of these.

A sedative is a drug which can reduce agitation and anxiety and induce a restful state. (Nembutal)

A hypnotic induces a state similar to natural sleep. (Seconal)

A tranquilizer relieves tension and anxiety without inducing drowsiness. (Sparine, Valium)

An analgesic reduces or eliminates pain without loss of consciousness. Analgesics may be swallowed or ingested (barbiturates, Demerol) or inhaled. (Nitrous oxide, Trilene)
An anesthetic induces loss of feeling with or without consciousness — regional or general. (Pudendal, epidural, paracervical)

Most women in North America are given one or several of these drugs in the course of labor. My own surveys of Montreal hospitals show that 85% of women have regional anesthesia, usually the continuous epidural block, in the first stage of labor. Furthermore, because of the practice of performing episiotomy routinely, 98% have regional anesthesia for second stage (expulsion). Many of these women also receive a sedative or analgesic earlier in labor.

In North America several decades ago, barbiturates were used routinely to relieve pain, general anesthesia then being given for delivery. The once-popular amnesic, scopolamine, has in most hospitals been discarded because of the undesirable restlessness and vocal activity often produced by the drug. Likewise, the famous "twilight sleep" has been replaced by regional anesthesia. But these two methods are still being used on occasion. Recently I discussed labor drugs with a pediatrician who works in the intensive care unit at a children's hospital. "You'd be amazed at the number of babies whose mothers were chock full of barbiturates!" she said. "I'm shocked at how much medication is being given in our city hospitals — even scopolamine is still used at some. Some babies come in with severe respiratory distress and it can be weeks before the full effects of the drugs have worn off."

Rarely are women given accurate information about possible side effects of drugs taken in labor; furthermore, my Montreal surveys indicate that only 30-40% of women attend any form of childbirth preparation class, to enable themselves to have an unmedicated birth. Yet, the late Dr. Virginia Apgar, world famous authority on birth defects and originator of the routinely used Apgar newborn evaluation chart, described the placenta not as a barrier, the frequently used term of description, but as a "bloody sieve". She stated that, "Almost everything ingested by or injected into the mother can be expected to reach the fetus within a few minutes."[14] One big hazard of childbirth drugs is oxygen deprivation. Many drugs depress the respiratory center of the brain, causing the baby to require resuscitation. Some sources estimate that as many as 60% of babies require resuscitation.[15.] (In one recent childbirth film designed for prenatal education, the mother — although she has an epidural forceps delivery — is described as having "natural childbirth". The use of the infant resuscitator on her child is shown, seemingly as the norm.)

Before birth, drugs are excreted by way of the mother's system. However, the newborn's body can't eliminate drugs so efficiently. The result of a drugged delivery is often a drowsy baby who sucks poorly. The drugs' effects can last several weeks — long enough to sabotage the mother's attempts to establish successful breastfeeding.

What about a *small* dose of drugs — not enough to cause respiratory distress; just enough to "take the edge off" as hospital staff promise. Unfortunately, it seems that even a minimal dose may affect the woman's control if she is using the Prepared Childbirth techniques. Dr. Vellay states flatly that the woman using psychoprophylaxis must avoid all brain depressants, because they will work against the principles vital to the method.

I have watched many times as both unprepared and prepared women were urged to have "just a little Demerol" in the hour or so before birth — but I've never heard anyone tell the mother of possible side effects. Demerol, a synthetic morphine, a barbiturate-type drug, is one of the more popular drugs in most hospitals. It reduces pain by relaxing muscles. It also appears to relax the cervix. Occasionally it produces euphoria. But Plantevin warns that respiratory distress to the infant may result if the drug if given one to three hours preceding delivery. [16] Boston University's Dr. Sumner Yaffe gives evidence to show that Demerol may not only affect respiration but learning and development for up to a month. "The ability to respond to stimuli and the learned inhibition of response were significantly decreased in treated infants." [17] Leading pediatrician T. Berry Brazelton describes similar observations. "Eight years ago, I was perplexed by many of the babies I saw in the nurseries of our lying-in hospitals. Each one had been sent to the nursery with an excellent Apgar score . . . but all too often as the nursery nurse made one of her frequent checks she found the infant, blue, cold, breathing shallowly, difficult to arouse. Although doctors are used to this sort of thing it is still very disturbing." [18]

Dr. N. J. Eastman, former editor of *Obstetrical and Gynecological Survey*, writes, "I am certain that any obstetrician with experience with sedative drugs would agree that the onset of respiration is usually less prompt and less vigorous when sedative drugs have been given than when they have been completely withheld." [19]

General anesthesia has in most areas been replaced by regional anesthetics. If a "general" is used, the popular "Trilene" is usually the choice, which does not appear to have a significant effect on the newborn.

Regional Anesthesia

In most major cities, local or regional anesthetics are the popular choice for childbirth. Commonly given are the epidural, paracervical and pudendal blocks.

Paracervical block is a local blocking of sensation of the nerves going to the uterus. Local analgesia is injected into either side of the cervix, by a needle inserted through the vagina. Sensation from contractions is reduced. It is not a painful procedure. Usually it is given in the hour before birth. Because it does not affect the perineum, it does not weaken the women's urge to push.

But it's not as harmless as it seems. Paracervical block has been found to cause slowing of the fetal heart rate (brachycardia). In 1968, Dr. H. R. Gordon published data showing that analgesia given by paracervical block is rapidly absorbed into the mother's blood circulation and crosses the placenta to reach the fetus about twenty minutes after administration.[20]

Pudendal block is local analgesia to the perineum just prior to delivery. It is usually used for episiotomy and frequently for forceps delivery. It usually impairs the "bearing down" reflex and the mother's control of the actual expulsion.

The Big E

". . . thus with this type of anesthetic you will be awake, will see the baby being born, will hear it cry and the baby will be born with no inhaling anesthetic.

In fact this is really natural childbirth of the best kind.

— from a pamphlet to expectant mothers distributed by a "family-centered" general hospital.

Epidural anesthesia is a precise procedure only undertaken by a skilled anesthetist. The woman is usually separated from her coach and moved to the delivery room, where she sits, bending forward, on the edge of the delivery table, supported by a nurse. A dose of analgesic drug is injected through the lower back into the epidural space outside the spine. Almost immediately, sensation is blocked from the waist down. Usually a fine tube, or catheter is inserted into the epidural space, brought up the woman's back and attached to a syringe which contains more of the drug for possible "top up" doses. The syringe is taped to the woman's shoulder. The process is not particularly uncomfortable unless a contraction begins as the epidural is given.

After the epidural the woman will cease to feel contraction sensations and may rest until delivery. In most cases, the loss of or impared sensation weakens or removes the woman's urge to push. A high percentage (about 75%) of epidural deliveries are performed with low forceps.

The epidural block necessitates close and constant supervision of the mother, because a fall in her blood pressure is a common result. "An intravenous infusion should always be set up prior to the establishment of the block and emergency resuscitation equipment must always be available," writes Dr. Odile Plantevin in *Analgesia and Anaesthesia in Obstetrics*. She explains that low blood pressure, the most frequent side effect of epidural, is aggravated if the woman lies on her back. It usually can be corrected if the woman rolls to one side. But if this low blood pressure is not recognized and treated it will reduce placental circulation, decrease uterine contractions, may endanger the mother's life and certainly harm the fetus.

She adds that, "The patient must never be left alone in the supine position and must not get out of bed as it would lead to marked pooling of blood in her legs and severe hypotension . . . Some degree of muscle weakness is often present, especially after repeated injections, and she may need help to move . . . The mother's blood pressure must be checked every five minutes during the first 20 minutes and every 30 minutes thereafter . . . the bladder will be insensitive and retention of urine may occur without the patient's being aware of it."[21]

I have watched busy nurses in rush hour try to carry out the frequent checks prescribed by Plantevin. More often, I have seen conditions far from ideal, caused simply by a case room staff overloaded with too many epidurals, done routinely.

At present the epidural appears to be the safest anesthetic with minimum effects on the baby. However, it is not true to say, as many doctors routinely tell their patients, that "The epidural has no effect on the baby." Research shows that all local anesthetics used in epidurals cross the placenta, and may depress the infant by drug effect or by lowering the mother's blood pressure.

One study indicates that the epidural can dramatically slow down the fetal heart rate — in at least 25% of fetuses whose mothers are administered this anesthetic in early labor.[22] Furthermore, studies by Burns and Gurtner, published in *Johns Hopkins Magazine*, suggest that any drug given during labor

— be it a sedative or regional anesthetic — may possibly affect the fetus. Their studies indicate that nearly all drugs have the potential of inhibiting the action of the oxygen-binding enzyme, Cytochrome P-450 — thus reducing oxygen transport to the baby via the placenta. Although more research in this area is needed, Burns' and Gurtner's report certainly indicates that the medical profession should use extreme caution in the use of the epidural and all other drugs in childbirth. [23]

Speaking in Ottawa recently, Dr. Murray Enkin said that the epidural not only can slow labor, but also depresses brain patterns in the fetus. The Big E's effects on infant reflexes and sucking responses can be observed for several days after birth, he said. For this reason, he strongly believes that the woman, not the doctor, should decide whether an epidural is necessary.

His observation is borne out by the research of K. Standley and colleagues — whose 1974 study indicates that the use of any local or regional anesthesia (such as the epidural or "paracervical block") can result in an irritable newborn with (temporarily) impaired motor control. 60 three-day-old infants were studied. The most alert, least irritable, and most mature in motor skills were those six babies whose mothers had not received analgesics or anesthetic. The remaining 54 showed decreased motor maturity and greater irritability, as indicated by jerky movements, crying, and a tendency to startle easily. The authors conclude: "Local-regional anesthetics . . . continue to be considered a safe choice in standard obstetric procedures. Our data raise questions about the assumption that routine usage . . . is inconsequential, even for the normal healthy infant." [24]

In 1969, my goddaughter, Clare was born at a city hospital. Her mother was given an epidural towards the end of labor. A few minutes after birth, Clare developed severe respiratory distress and was rushed to a children's intensive care unit where she remained for two weeks.

"The pediatrician told me that there was little hope that

Clare would live," says her mother. "In fact, he asked me to sign an autopsy consent form. He was quite frank and said the epidural could have caused the problem — my blood pressure had been low."

But Clare survived — a miracle, said her doctor. Month after month, both terrified parents watched for signs of damage — over-reacting to coughs and colds, unable to relax and enjoy their baby until her developmental milestones proved she was normal. I attended the birth of Clare's baby brother — this one totally unmedicated — and shared the parents' joy as their pink healthy son was born. Perhaps this is an extreme example, but Clare's mother's obstetrician now believes that epidural should only be used when absolutely necessary.

So does Sandra H., mother of four school-aged children, who was one of the earlier women to use the Big E:

> *When my first child was born, my obstetrician told me about the epidural — "painless, natural childbirth", he called it, and I was thrilled. During the labor, they told me to tell them when it hurt. I dutifully reported each twinge and they kept me topped up throughout. It was painless, all right — but for several days afterward, I could barely breathe or walk or get out of bed.*
>
> *I used PC for my other three children — and in all cases, I felt fine afterwards. My three younger children are extremely bright, but the eldest has a learning disability. I can't tell you how many times I've wondered if that heavy dosage of epidural — probably more than I needed — was responsible for his problems in school.*

Sandra H. and her child may well have been the victims of epidural overdose. If epidural is deemed absolutely necessary because of a complicated labor, it should be given minimally, in *late labor only*, by a skilled anesthetist, supported by careful nursing care. Under such controlled conditions, a Boston research team recently studied the effects of minimal analgesia and anesthesia on newborns, following the babies through the first ten days of life. Their study indicates that all analgesics and regional anesthetics — including the epidural — affect the fetus to some degree. But when given under ideal conditions, these effects can be minimal and short-lasting — particularly in the case of epidural. The authors conclude, "Our results do seem to be reassuring to mothers who either choose to or are forced by circumstances to have a minimal, well-controlled amount of analgesic premedication or anesthesia."[25]

In 1967, I watched the early epidurals being used in Montreal. They were then used only for difficult labors because of possible side effects, and the skill required to give them. Three years later, "the Big E" had become routine, and is now used on close to 80% of all deliveries. I have watched the epidural relieve pain and suffering in the unprepared woman and in cases of difficult labors. Few people would argue that suffering is better in this case. But if the woman is well prepared to handle labor without epidural, the hospital atmosphere will probably discourage her attempt to do so.

"I just didn't need anything," Jan told me, "but I was certainly tempted. The nurse told me almost as soon as I arrived that most women needed epidural and she didn't see the point in suffering. She told me I'd better have it soon or it would be too late."

"We now know that there is a 5-10% chance of post epidural headache," says Miriam, "We didn't know that when our first child was born. I had top-up doses several times even though I had not been in pain. My doctor said he didn't believe in suffering, but I suffered for two weeks afterwards from a sore back and severe headaches."

The epidural generally slows contractions, so induction may be required to speed things up. The use of stirrups for expulsion becomes mandatory. Forceps and episiotomy tend to become routine because of impaired sensation. To describe the epidural as "natural childbirth of the best kind" is not only untrue, but absurd. The only "natural" aspect is that the woman is awake.

Verbal Anesthesia — Why Not?

It is the mother who must ultimately bear the major emotional burden of a damaged or impaired child. Under normal conditions, no one should usurp the mother's prerogative by placing her unborn or newborn infant at a possible disadvantage without her consent . . . In the light of the frequent scientific papers being published now on this possible hazards resulting from the use of regional anesthesia, it would seem prudent to make every effort to prepare the mother physically and mentally to cope with the sensations and discomfort of birth in order to avoid the use of such medicaments.

—Doris Haire.[26]

In France and the Netherlands, childbirth drugs are reserved for complicated or operative deliveries. In Holland, where more than 80% of women are prepared for childbirth with breathing and relaxation techniques, fewer than 5% of women require drugs. But in most of North America, fewer than 40% are prepared in any way for labor and about 85% of women are given drugs.

The United States has more infant deaths due to birth injuries and respiratory distress than any other developed country; there is growing concern over the rapid increase in children with "learning disabilities". In the light of recent research, obstetrical medication plays a significant part in such neurological disability. The high percentage of drugged deliveries is not entirely the fault of medical personnel, however. As one nurse told me, "We have dozens of women who come in, and right away they're asking when they can have an epidural."

I have coached many unprepared women through labor. Despite the lack of preparation, very few of these women needed medication, when given constant support and encouragement. I strongly believe that childbirth drugs should be reserved for difficult labors. Every woman should be given the opportunity to prepare physically and psychologically for labor; every woman should be "coached" and supported throughout labor; and verbal analgesia should be used before drugs are deemed necessary.

The "Delivery" Room

I think the worst part was when I started to feel like pushing. They wheeled me down the hall into the delivery room and I had to wriggle onto the table. Just as I was halfway on I had a contraction and I was sure the IV was going to pull out. My husband was off changing, my doctor wasn't there and I knew the baby was coming. I kept yelling for my husband and the doctor, but all they told me was, "Don't push — your doctor's on his way." They seemed more concerned about getting me strapped into stirrups and covering me up than about how I was feeling. The baby's head was right there when the doctor finally made it . . .

— Susan G.

For most women, the contractions just prior to the delivery stage are the most intense and difficult to control. Most women become totally absorbed with the body and become extremely sensitive to any interruption or interference. The transfer to delivery room at the end of this phase causes a large degree of disturbance and probably anxiety. Complaining about this routine, Alice C., whose hobby is breeding dogs, says angrily, "My vet told me that the worst thing you can do for a bitch in labor is to move her. Why haven't doctors caught on that it's the same for human mothers?"

In the hospital I worked at in Northern Ontario, I often watched nurses cross the woman's legs to hold back the baby until the doctor arrived. Fortunately this cruel practice is no longer in use — neither is the hospital — but little has been done to dispel the anxiety of the woman who is told that her baby cannot be born until the doctor arrives. "Please hurry, Doctor, I can't wait any longer!" is an anguished cry I've heard countless times.

Doris Haire cites one study where the labors of mice were disturbed by noises, lights and moving from one box to another during labor. Labor was as much as 72% longer and 54% more mouse pups were born dead than in the undisturbed control group.[27]
Leading sociologist and childbirth educator, Niles Newton, in "Effects of Environmental Disturbances in Labor", concludes that if a mouse is so disturbed, the far more highly developed nervous system of the human may be equally sensitive to environmental differences in labor. And a recent study of monkeys finds that maternal psychological stress can cause breathing difficulty in the infant.[28] These studies suggest that hospital labors with their noise, lights, questionnaires, examinations, equipment and moving may cause undesirable side-effects by increasing anxiety in the laboring woman.

In most European countries, obstetrical personnel understand the importance of a calm, unhurried, childbirth atmosphere. Women remain in one room for the entire course of labor, delivery and the initial hours after birth. This practice eliminates stress for the mother, and spares the nurse the problem of deciding when to transfer the woman to the delivery room — leaving her free to support and encourage the woman.

Supine Birth Position

I was perfectly in control. I asked if I could sit up and push without stirrups. Everyone was horrified and before I could protest, they had me flat on my back, my legs in stirrups, my hands in handcuffs, my lower half was covered with yards of draping.
                                                              —*Elsie E.*

Until a few years ago in Montreal, many hospitals required each woman, regardless of whether she was medicated or not, to push lying flat. They discouraged her efforts to pull head and shoulders up to round the spine and adopt a more comfortable pushing position. Before fathers were included at the birth, a nurse might support the woman's head and shoulders. When I coached, in the delivery room, supporting the women became my job. But numerous women who took my classes reported that nobody helped them — indeed, some doctors told them to lie down flat and push.

At a convention of The International Childbirth Education Association in Milwaukee, 1972, a roar of delighted laughter broke out when one speaker suggested that any doctor who required a woman to deliver flat on her back (lithotomy position) should first be required to have a bowel movement in the position. He went one step further: prospective obstetricians should be required to write their exams with an IV set up!

Only in North America is the lithotomy position used routinely for birth. In most other countries women squat, or use a semi-sitting or side-lying (Sim's) position. These positions allow the spine to be curved (the easiest position for birthing) and permit the woman to work with rather than against the pull of gravity. In Sweden, a table with a tilted back is used. Recently a similar table, the "birth couch" was introduced in North America, but few hospitals have been "radical" enough to buy it.

Like the immobile position required for monitoring, the supine birth position can cause fetal distress, according to Dr. Caldeyro-Barcia. He maintains that when the woman lies on her back, the pressure on the large blood vessels around the heart causes a drop in the mother's blood pressure and reduced oxygen supply to the baby. He believes that the best labor position is walking, followed closely by side-lying or sitting.[29]

Lithotomy position not only puts undue pressure upon blood vessels, but also upon the back. The woman works tremendously hard against gravity; the rigid position in which the stirrups hold her legs puts tension on the perineum and *maximizes* the possibility of tearing.

Episiotomy
With my first baby I had no choice but to have episio-

*tomy: my doctor did them routinely. The repair hurt —
the doctor was instructing an intern and it seemed to
take longer than the birth. It hurt for weeks after. I told
the doctor and he said, "Funny, it usually doesn't." He
made me feel like a hypochondriac!
I had so much pain I didn't want to make love ever
again. When we finally did, I was tense and afraid that
the incision would rip open. It was so painful that our
sex life was a disaster for months after.
For my second child I went looking for a doctor who
didn't do episiotomy routinely. I got all the stock answers about having all my organs fall out later and not
enjoying sex. Finally I found a doctor who agreed to try
to avoid episiotomy if possible. I practised pelvic floor
exercises every day and during the birth I didn't use stirrups. The doctor seemed to ease the head out very slowly and I controlled the pushing. I managed not to tear. I
could walk around the next day and start to enjoy my
baby . . . the difference it made to our sexual relationship was unbelievable.*

—Lisa P.

One advertisement in a medical magazine supports the idea
of pain with episiotomy: "Baby's Fine — but Mother Still
Hurts . . . after episiotomy or cesarean section, Empirin with
codeine every four hours will help make mother more
comfortable!"

"I don't know what you women are fussing about — it's
only a small incision and it's not painful," doctors are always
telling me. But I have seen enough, from my work on maternity floors to know they are incorrect. I have watched countless women struggle through the first day, unable to sit comfortably, shuffling with legs apart, telling me, as we try positions and exercises to relieve pain, "The stitches were the
worst part."

Few doctors deny the stress of the days after birth. Physically, the mother is recovering from loss of blood and normal

labor stress; her breasts may be uncomfortable and her nipples sore, particularly if hospital schedules have withheld her baby for many hours at first. Psychologically, she must adjust to the role of mothering. She must wear sanitary pads to absorb the vaginal discharge, "lochia", which follows birth and lasts several weeks. The itching of new hair growth following a shave is uncomfortable. One more "minor discomfort" looms large at this time.

Yet episiotomy is performed in 98% of all births in many areas. Obstetricians rationalize that it prevents:

1. Tearing (a clean surgical incision is better than a large ragged tear).
2. Neurological damage to the baby from lengthy delivery.
3. Weakness of the perineum in later life.
4. Loss of sexual enjoyment (his and hers).

Currently there is some controversy whether episiotomy should be "median" or "mediolateral". The median incision — less uncomfortable for the woman — runs in a straight line below the vagina, but there is a slight risk of cutting the anal sphincter. The mediolateral runs outwards towards the thigh. This avoids problems with the anal sphincter but it is frequently extremely painful for the woman. Stitches can become infected and many women experience slow healing.

I haven't been able to find much evidence that the four cited reasons for routine episiotomy have validity. For example, "tearing" is a rarity if the delivery is handled properly. In Holland and France, where less than 20% of women require episiotomy, I watched several women deliver their first babies. No episiotomy was performed and no tearing occurred.

A well-known British midwife, Chloe Fisher believes that tearing can be prevented in most cases by letting the woman find a comfortable position, and providing supportive staff and a calm, relaxed atmosphere. "If the patient is lying flat on her back, she has an almost impossible task to perform and will tire more rapidly," she states. She stresses the need for more exercises to make the perineum more elastic and teach control of the muscles. In countries where episiotomy is not routine, such exercises are taught every woman, before and after birth.[30]

I believe that obstetricians might have a tough time proving that episiotomy reduces neurological impairment to the baby. Doris Haire cites the example of 17,000 children, all born in the same week in Great Britain and followed up for seven years. Her statistics indicate that a second stage of labor lasting as long as two and one half hours does not increase the incidence of neurological impairment for the full term infant who shows no fetal distress.[31]

And I can't find any evidence that episiotomy prevents weakened organs and muscles later in life; in contrast, there seems to be some evidence that episiotomy can cause permanent physical and emotional damage. Because episiotomy itself cuts through not only muscle, but nerves and blood vessels, loss of sensation frequently results. British anthropologist and childbirth educator, Sheila Kitzinger observes that an intact perineum maintained by post partum-exercises minimizes problems in sexual enjoyment for both man and woman — more so than a perineum which is surgically cut and repaired. "The episiotomy may be conceptualized as a sexual attack and especially if the delivery has been by forceps, birth can be seen by the woman as a sort of rape." She adds that women suffering from poor episiotomy repair may suffer entrance dyspareunia (spasm upon entrance) on sexual intercourse.[32]

France's Dr. Pierre Vellay told a meeting of the Montreal Childbirth Education Association that he does not see the need for episiotomy routinely. "If the woman is pushing well and if the doctor is patient there is usually no problem." His films of birth showed his controlled deliveries: he applies counter pressure to the perineum and eases the head out, with not a tear. As the film finished I heard a doctor sitting near me mutter to his friend, "God — they're all going to come in and ask for that now!"

The techniques to avoid tearing need practice, however. Unfortunately, few medical doctors or students have watched birth without episiotomy. Epidural has made forceps almost routine, and their use requires episiotomy. But for most women, merely anticipating the procedure creates anxiety.

The Rise of Caesarean Birth

As the managed birth has become the norm, the Caesarean birth rate has climbed steadily, from 4-6% in 1974 to a current 12-15% in North America. A rate of 20-30% is not uncommon in large hospitals.

The Caesarean birth undeniably has a place in obstetrical care. Certainly the procedure is safer than it has even been, but it remains a procedure not without side effects for mother and baby. It is, after all, major surgery.

Increased maternal risks include pain and complications associated with major surgery; prolonged post-surgical disability; interruption of mother-infant attachment; and maternal psychological disturbances. According to one report, the incidence of post-surgical complications (hemorrhage, infection, and the like) in Caesarean mothers, is reported to be almost 50%.[33]

Moreover, the increasing Caesarean birthrate has not been shown to produce healthier newborns. The Banta-Thacker report for the U.S. National Health Services suggests that the value of electronic fetal monitoring and Caesarean section in preventing brain damage is purely spectulative.[34]

Why then are numbers of Caesarean births increasing dramatically? According to the Banta-Thacker report, "The complex causes for the rise in Caesarean section include cephalopelvic disproportion (CPD), breech, fetal distress, repeat Caesarean, alterations in residency training programs, the more interventionistic stance of the obstetric community, and (italics mine) *the financial incentives which may encourage Caesarean section.*" (In the U.S., cost is about three times greater for a Caesarean than a vaginal birth.)

The report suggests that half the rise in the Caesarean rate could be attributed to electronic fetal monitoring, and thereby, one would assume, fetal distress.

But if we examine the ingredients of a routinely managed labor, we see many factors which may contribute to fetal distress. Procedures which produce anxiety may slow the progress of labor and also decrease the oxygen flow to the unborn child. The artificial rupture of membranes in early labor, restricting a woman's mobility; the routine glucose IV, oxytoxics and anesthesia are all procedures which, research indicates, may also contribute to fetal distress.

I believe that parents who are prepared to work with labor, and who are able to make informed decisions about labor management, are less likely to have a Caesarean birth. In thirteen years, I have prepared more than five thousand couples in childbirth education programs. The Caesarean birth rate has remained at about 6%, despite the fact that many of the women in my classes are defined as "high-risk".

I attribute this low rate to the fact that the prepared woman is more likely to remain mobile, to avoid unnecessary hospital procedures, and to minimize the need for drugs in childbirth. Today, there is a rapid growth in support groups for Caesarean parents. While I agree that such groups are vitally needed, I believe that the medical community must examine closely the factors contributing to the soaring surgical birth rate.

Management of the Placenta

Maternal medication and early clamping of the cord can cause difficulty in the third stage of labor — expulsion of the placenta. The uterus may be sluggish and unable to contract sufficiently to expel the "afterbirth". As a result, as soon as the baby is born, hospitals routinely give the mother a shot of the hormone oxytocin, which is used in induction, to stimulate uterine contractions. So effective is this drug that the placenta follows the baby in the next ten minutes or so — allowing the doctor to get to work repairing the episiotomy.

On many occasions, I've watched obstetricians speed up expulsion of the placenta even more, by pulling on the umbilical cord — a practice which some authorities believe is a common cause of hemorrhage.[36] And I have spoken with many women who have experienced problems in this stage of labor. Some developed excessive bleeding in the hours following birth; others were forced to return to hospital after they had been discharged, with suspected retention of a fragment of the placenta which required a "D & C" (dilation and curettage of the uterus) — minor surgery, requiring further hospitalization. When I discussed the births, each woman remembered that the doctor seemed to pull on the cord, and the placenta came away rapidly.

In European countries where oxytocin is not given, where medication rate is low and cords are clamped after three or four minutes, problems with the placenta are rare. It is regarded as normal for the placenta to take as long as thirty minutes to come away. And of course no episiotomy repair is usually necessary, because episiotomy is not routine in Europe.

Recently I watched one case where haste seemed the theme. As soon as the (nonmedicated) baby was out, the cord was cut and clamped without ever putting the infant on the mother's abdomen. The baby was taken to the side of the room, and the doctor started to push on the mother's abdomen and pull on the cord. "If it doesn't come soon we'll have to give you some gas and go in and get it," he told the mother, who had worked with labor with no medication but now winced in pain. Five minutes later the placenta arrived. Only ten minutes had elapsed since the birth. A few minutes for the episiotomy repair and the doctor was off. Total time he'd spent in the delivery room was 35 minutes.

These routines are common to most North American births, with few modifications and exceptions. (Another unfortunate hospital routine — that of routinely separating mother and baby, will be discussed in detail in Chapter 10.) Like tinkering with the environment, obstetrical interference becomes a vicious chain or circle, creating more problems which require still more technology.

Childbirth is viewed as an illness — by most obstetrical personnel on this continent. This, to me, is the heart of the problem. Doctors and nurses pass on this notion to the women they consider to be sick "patients" rather than healthy "clients". As a result, few women have the opportunity to experience childbirth as a joyous, natural event; only a minority are adequately prepared to work with their bodies in labor.

The unprepared woman requires pain relief, particularly if she is not given adequate "verbal sedation". Thus, heavy reliance on anesthetics is viewed as part of "normal" labor. Anesthesia interrupts the natural rhythms of labor: it needs elaborate equipment to monitor and regulate; IV's and inductions to speed up what anesthesia slows down. It needs a move to a "delivery room"; supports for legs which are heavy from anesthetic; episiotomy to widen the outlet for the forceps which are required because the woman can't push effectively. It often requires acceleration of the birth in order to resuscitate the baby; hormones to hasten the placenta — which would normally be expelled by the sucking of the baby at breast — hurrying the episiotomy repair as quickly as possible. Too often the result is a mother and baby who are far from *well* — and childbirth indeed becomes an illness.

It should not be forgotten, however, that many of these technological advances in obstetrics have saved the lives of mothers and babies who otherwise would have died. I certainly do not object to their use in the high-risk delivery. I do, however, protest their routine use for births without complication — about 90% of all labors. But regardless of degree of risk in her childbirth, each woman should have access to the *other* developments in obstetrics that have been made in this century. By "other", I refer to the great humanitarian discoveries regarding the non-medical relief of pain in childbirth — the work of people such as Britain's Grantly Dick-Read, France's Fernand Lamaze and Pierre Vellay, Elisabeth Bing of the U.S.A., and Dr. Murray Enkin in Canada — which will be outlined in the following chapter.

4 Revolution in the delivery room

In 1967 I became Charge Physiotherapist at the Catherine Booth Hospital in Montreal, then a woman's hospital which thousands of couples fondly remember as a warm, personal place to have a baby — a pioneer in true "family-centered maternity care" in Canada. For fifteen years, two physiotherapists had been offering an excellent prenatal program at the hospital — one of the first in the city. The course, based on the teachings of Grantly Dick-Read, included a tremendously popular "orientation" evening for fathers.

Young and single, I was not particularly excited by the idea of prenatal work, and viewed the job as a temporary stop on my way to Europe. But after all, it was my job. I began to watch births, talk to women and learn everything I could about childbirth.

After a little research, I learned that the North American way of birth is rooted in a well-intentioned movement to improve woman's lot in childbirth. The concept of childbirth as painful and potentially dangerous has its origins in Biblical times. The legendary "Eve's Curse" of Genesis 3:16, "In sorrow thou shalt bring forth children..." has been interpreted down through history as "in pain and suffering" for most women. Other Biblical passages such as Isaiah 13:8, "They shall be in pain as a woman that travailleth," have reinforced the traditional view of the curse of childbirth. Moreover, until recently, birth was a time of great risk for both mother and baby: hygiene standards were poor, infection was rampant, attendants frequently inexpert. As a result, many women and babies died in childbirth.

Until the reign of Louis XIV, most European women used the "birthing stool" which originated in Roman times. With this "stool" — a horseshoe shaped chair with hollow centre — the woman was able to birth in a comfortable position, leaning forward, assisted by gravity, the birth area discreetly concealed. According to history, Louis delighted in watching his mistresses give birth — concealed behind a curtain. (He was perhaps the earliest "father in the delivery room" on record at such a formal birth!) To allow him a better view, he convinced the court physician to popularize a high table, the forerunner of the modern delivery table. The woman gave birth lying on her back: delivery, although easier for attendant and observer, became more difficult for the woman required to push against gravity. Comfort was sacrificed to fashion and the birthstool gradually became obsolete.

By the early nineteenth century, maternity hospitals were beginning to appear in Europe. In 1847, at the Allegemeines Krankenhaus in Vienna, Dr. Ignaz Philipp Semmelweis discovered that puerperal fever — the deadly bacterial infection which swept through maternity wards — could be virtually eliminated by aseptic conditions. As a result, "childbed fever" was reduced by nine-tenths. At the same time, Britain's James Simpson was using chloroform to relieve pain in childbirth. Chloroform was at first regarded with suspicion, but after Queen Victoria delivered her sixth son, Prince Leopold, under its influence, its use became fashionable — and it was followed by the use of other pain-relieving medications.

North America followed European obstetrical practices. As forceps techniques became more highly developed, and anesthesia more routine, doctors began to replace midwives. In medical schools, obstetrics became a rapidly expanding specialty. Anesthesia, forceps and asepsis (use of sterile gloves, clothing and birth equipment) could best be utilized in a hospital, and most skilfully administered by doctors.

At the turn of the century, conflict arose between the midwives and the group of obstetricians so readily replacing them. Obstetricians denounced and ridiculed midwives as "hopelessly dirty, ignorant and incompetent." In *Witches, Midwives and Nurses,* Barbara Ehrenreich and Deirdre English relate that midwives were "held accountable for the prevalence of uterine infections and neo-natal blindness due to parental infection from gonorrhea, two conditions easily preventable by hand washing to prevent the former, eye drops the latter." Midwives retaliated by accusing obstetricians of being "too ready to use surgical techniques which endangered mother and child." At the turn of the century in the United States, women were spending approximately five million dollars per year on midwives' fees — fees which were coveted by the new class of "professionals." The medical profession lobbied for government legislation to outlaw the midwife. Gradually she became illegal throughout the United States and Canada, and the obstetrician gained a monopoly on childbirth. In 1910, about 50% of North American births were home-delivered by midwives. Forty years later, 86% were hospital-born, and 95% of babies were delivered by physicians. The doctor-hospital pattern of childbirth had become rigidly established.[1]

With the decline of midwifery, childbirth became male-dominated as well as hospital-centered. The woman entering the hospital was now cut off from all that was familiar and warm. If she was lucky, she would have her husband with her for part of the labor. If not, she would endure the hours alone, broken only by visits from the nurse or doctor to check the progress of labor.

The hospital shave and enema, to facilitate hygiene standards of hospital birth, became rituals to be somehow undergone as quickly as possible, and were faced with fear and apprehension by many women. The medication, administered for humane reasons, caused drowsiness — or in the case of the once popular drug, "scopolamine," other undesirable side effects. One 1974 textbook of obstetrics advises that where scopolamine is used, "constant supervision is mandatory as various degrees of excitement, physical and vocal activity, hallucinations and even delirium occur with this medication." (Recently, I was astounded to learn that this drug is still used.) Other painkillers, when combined with scopolamine, caused amnesia. To cope with "physical and vocal activity," women were usually restrained by having the sides of the labor bed raised. With the woman reduced to a twilight state of muffled pain and drowsiness, the father could do little to help. Suffering mental anguish, he became almost relieved when asked to wait outside when the woman was ready to give birth.

Asepsis, anesthesia, forceps and other instruments are best used in a bright, sterile room, similar to an operating theatre. So, at a time when labor is most stressful, and comfort and reassurance imperative for her emotional well-being, the woman was moved from the labor bed to a cold, harsh delivery room.

Once in the delivery area, she was given a variation of chloroform, sometimes combined with ether to give "twilight sleep." Unable to co-operate, and very likely in a state of uncontrollable "physical and vocal activity," she was placed in a position convenient for the obstetrician. She lay on a narrow table which reached only to her buttocks, because forceps and episiotomy are best performed with the doctor in front. Her legs were strapped out of the way and held wide apart by metal stirrups, and her flailing hands were confined by leather handcuffs.

Because of this position (lithotomy), the effects of

medication and the woman's resulting inability to co-operate, episiotomy (incision of the perineum) became necessary to prevent tearing. The episiotomy was also performed to shorten the length of time the baby spent in the vagina and to facilitate use of forceps. Because the medication administered to the mother rapidly crossed the placenta and caused fetal depression, the doctor needed to get the child out quickly. Forceps, introduced to save lives in complicated births, became routinely used in order to speed up the passage of the baby. Sterile "drapes" over the woman's legs and a brilliant spotlight completed the picture of a "sick" female patient in a hospital operating theatre — rather than that of a healthy woman performing a normal biological function.

After the child was born, the umbilical cord was clamped immediately — partly to lessen the amount of medication passed to the infant. Many babies needed resuscitation, and were unable to suck strongly at the breast — nor was the woman in any state to offer it. The baby was assigned to a specially trained nursery staff who simulated natural feeding as best as they could with glucose and water and formula. Artificial feeding became popular, promoted by a rapidly-growing baby-food industry: as well as being the new hygienic way to feed, mothers were told, it gave them freedom from the home.

The mother's recovery was slow. She was not strong enough to care for her child: this was done by the hospital staff. Gradually her milk supply dwindled and artificial feeding became inevitable. Finally the couple left the hospital, uneasy with the small stranger and with each other. Ill-prepared for the demanding job of parenthood, they became totally reliant on advice from "experts", finding comfort in strict adherence to schedules and rules. As a result, their decision-making and confidence were undermined from the beginning.

Today, general anesthesia is rarely used, replaced by regional forms such as the epidural. Although these appear to have minimal effects on mother and baby — as I have explained in Chapter 3 — many studies indicate that they are not without risk. As a result of the new local anesthetics, most women today are awake and able to co-operate during birth. A large percentage of women and their partners are prepared in some way for labor. In addition, rapidly growing numbers of women are eager and fully able to breastfeed as soon as possible after birth.

Yet the old practices are slow to change. Delivery position remains basically unchanged, although a few hospitals modify it slightly to allow the woman to raise her head and shoulders and flex her spine for pushing. Stirrups are still regulation equipment — as are handcuffs in many hospitals. Episiotomy is performed in more than 90% of North American births.

Fragmented maternity care has become the norm — a group of specialists for the mother, another medical team for her baby. In many cases, the father is still treated as an outsider. Rules and regulations are still too often based on the needs of a bottle-fed infant, with little provision for the breastfeeding mother.

Natural Childbirth

At first, the best solution to pain in childbirth seemed to most doctors — and most women — to be blocking or deadening of sensation by childbirth drugs. By the early nineteen hundreds most women in Britain and other Western countries were giving birth under "twilight sleep." But while medicine was developing more techniques for the high-risk woman in childbirth — and undeniably cutting maternal and infant death rates — another approach to childbirth began to evolve, exploring the possibility of non-medical relief of pain in childbirth.

In 1914, English physician Grantly Dick-Read questioned whether pain in childbirth was inevitable. He began to try to reduce — or even eliminate — the pain before it began. While assisting a poor London woman during the birth of her child, he was impressed with her calm dignity. He offered her chloroform. She refused and afterward told him, "It didn't hurt. It wasn't meant to, was it doctor?"

After observing many women, Read concluded that the women who were most afraid experienced most pain; those who seemed calm appeared to have less. In 1933, in *Natural Childbirth,* he formulated the "fear-tension-pain" theory. Referring to the work of Russian scientist Pavlov — and his research in 1927 with dogs and the conditioned reflex — Read decided that women were socially conditioned to fear childbirth. The accumulation of verbal cues from historical tales and those of friends and relatives ("I'll never go through that again!") led them to expect pain and suffering. Fear produced muscular tension which in turn lowered the pain threshold. Early sensations were interpreted by the woman as "pain" and the vicious circle began. In 1944, Read wrote in *Childbirth Without Fear,* "I began to realize that there is no law in nature and no design which could justify the pain of childbirth."

With physiotherapist Helen Heardman, Read set up a program aimed at eliminating fear and thus pain. In *A Way to Natural Childbirth,* Heardman defines "natural childbirth" as being attained "when on the physical plane, labor is physiological and unobstructed, and on the mental plane the mother is unafraid, reaching the climax of the actual birth fully conscious, confident and joyous."

The classes, in Pavlovian terms, "deconditioned" women by knowledge and education, and further equipped them with physical fitness, relaxation and breathing control. The new "Natural Childbirth" — a term relevant at a time when childbirth had become truly "unnatural" by any definition — offered women a chance to participate in childbirth with dignity. The Read method also reduced the need for medication. But, unfortunately, this aspect was magnified out of proportion, by women and hospital staffs alike, and in many minds "Natural Childbirth" became synonymous with non-medicated childbirth and the notion of bravely suffering women.

Read admitted the problem, writing in *Childbirth Without Fear (1944):*

> *Women trained and prepared for a natural birth have suffered severe frustration and disappointment when deviation from the absolute normal is deemed best to be rectified by assistance. Others who suffered more discomfort than they were led to understand might occur have hesitated to ask for, and even been unwilling to receive, pain relief, and thereby increased their babies' and their own problems. Women improperly prepared believe that pain relief by injections, drugs or analgesics is evidence of failure and become morbidly depressed.*

Helen Heardman stresses in her book,

> *It is not often that anesthesia will be required, but it must be available and offered, though never forced, at the usual indications. The choice lies with the mother herself.*

Regrettably, many women appear to have fallen into the "improperly prepared" category, and "Natural Childbirth" took on overtones of martyrdom among some hospital staffs. It seems that Read's presence at labor contributed to the effectiveness of his principles. His method has been criticized as too empirical — based on observation rather than scientific knowledge — but he pioneered the way for other developments in the field of childbirth education and his method has benefited and continues to benefit thousands of women. In 1949, the Read method was adopted by the Maternity Center Association of New York. Today it is widely used in Britain, Australia, Canada, United States and New Zealand.

In 1947, Colorado physician Robert Bradley adopted Read's principles and later broadened the approach to "husband-coached" childbirth. Bradley, believing birth to be an important growth in the love of a man and woman, began to include the father as "coach". Author of *Husband-Coached Childbirth*, 1965, he is the founder of The American Academy Of Husband Coached Childbirth, which stresses the importance of non-medicated childbirth. Out of the 10,000 births which he has attended, 96.4% were non-medicated.

When I became a childbirth educator in 1967, the Read method was widely used in Canada. Read's teachings had been reinforced in 1956 by Dr. Attlee of Halifax in his book *Natural Childbirth* and at the Catherine Booth Hospital the method had flourished for fifteen years. Using Read's principles, I began to live in the hospital residence, coaching as many women as I could, day and night. The Read method was extremely helpful to almost every woman in early labor, I noticed. But when contractions became extremely strong, many women forgot what to do — unless a well trained coach was present.

In early 1968 I read Marjorie Karmel's *Thank you, Dr. Lamaze* and became excited at the idea of conditioned activity and the positive attitude which viewed childbirth in much the same way as an athletic event. Above all, I was impressed by the role of the "monitrice" — the physiotherapist who instructed the Karmels in the method during pregnancy and "coached" during labor and birth, providing extra encouragement for the couple. I investigated the method further.

Psychoprophylaxis (The Lamaze Method)

While Read was working on Natural Childbirth, a group of Russian scientists were also developing a method of reducing pain in childbirth. Based also on Pavlov's work, their method aimed at deconditioning the fear response to childbirth, but carried Read's approach one step further.

The Russians believed that if a woman could be conditioned to fear birth, and deconditioned not to fear it, she could be reconditioned to respond to labor sensations positively. The woman learned to respond to positive verbal cues, using controlled exercises practised repeatedly in a consistent pattern in the last weeks of pregnancy — until she was able to perform them almost without thought. The exercises, based on the conditioned reflex and cortical inhibition of the brain, conserved energy while giving her activity in response to uterine contractions. This "conscious controlled activity" involved neuromuscular control, controlled breathing patterns and other concentration tools such as light abdominal massage and a "concentration point" (usually fixed to a nearly wall). The method, termed "psychoprophylaxis" or "mind prevention" of pain, was so successful that it was adopted as the national method of childbirth by both Russia and later, China.

In 1951, sixty-year-old French obstetrician Fernand Lamaze travelled Russia and was greatly impressed by the use of prophylaxis which he witnessed. The following year, he introduced these principles into his practice at the Metal Workers' Clinic in Paris, adding a "fast breathing" technique and several other modifications. "A woman learns how to give birth in the same way that she learns to swim, or write or read, and she does so without pain," Lamaze wrote in his 1956 book, *Painless Childbirth*. He points out that total painlessness can be achieved only if medical staff sticks closely to the ground rules. "The attitude towards the parturient during pregnancy and labor is vitally important. The following are necessary: medical changes in the choice of words, hence altering their own vocabulary; finding the enthusiasm and energy which must permeate the method."

In 1959, a young American woman, Marjorie Karmel, wrote *Thank you, Dr. Lamaze*, describing the excitement of a painless birth at Château Belvedere near Paris under the guidance of Dr. Lamaze and his monitrice Mme Cohen. She then tells of her difficulty locating a doctor in New York who would "permit" her to use the method for her second child's birth. She went shopping for a doctor, encountered hostility and disbelief, but finally gave birth to her child by her chosen method. Her article in a national magazine drew attention to the Lamaze Method; and physiotherapist Elisabeth Bing arranged to meet Karmel.

Together, they set up classes in New York to teach psychoprophylaxis, and in 1960 Bing, together with medical professionals, founded ASPO (the American Society for Psychoprophylaxis in Obstetrics) which dedicates itself to the Lamaze Method, training teachers and arranging classes. In an effort to eliminate the unfavorable attitude to "natural childbirth," the ASPO introduced the term "Prepared Childbirth." And rather than stressing "no medication", the group emphasized the total physical, emotional and mental preparation of the woman in childbirth.

Prepared Childbirth

Using the Lamaze Method, I started coaching as many couples from my classes as I could, spending weeks at a time living in the hospital residence in order to be on hand at night. The results were tremendously exciting. I noticed that the presence of a "coach" gave the couple more confidence — but the man was still more of a bystander than a participant.

During the couples' evenings, the interest and enthusiasm of the men became apparent. They wanted to learn more about what they could do at home. I opened up all of the classes to the fathers.

It became obvious to me that the best person to coach is one who cares deeply about her — and the person who cares most deeply is usually the father. To be successful, a coach requires both a knowledge of the preparation techniques and time to build up rapport and function with the woman as a team. I began to include the father in every aspect of preparation, instructing him in coaching techniques.

Nothing is more powerful than a good idea whose time has come. This is true of husband-coached childbirth. Throughout North America other childbirth educators were also concluding that the father is the best coach. In many areas the teachers at first followed the European "monitrice" plan, coaching women themselves. Eventually, however, the sheer numbers of women wanting coached childbirth caused a problem — other coaches were needed. The father was welcomed as coach, and childbirth educators were delighted with the support and encouragement uniquely his.

In 1964, Dr. Murray Enkin introduced psychoprophylactic childbirth preparation classes to St. Joseph's Hospital, Hamilton, Ontario and pioneered a well co-ordinated team approach to couple oriented childbirth at this hospital. I consider Dr. Enkin to be the father of the couple-oriented birth movement in Canada. His influence has been enormous throughout the country, and under his guidance, St. Joseph's Hospital and McMaster Medical Centre have paved the way for other "family centered" units across the country.

In 1966, psychoprophylaxis received a boost from New York obstetrician Irwin Chabon in *Awake and Aware — Participating In Childbirth Through Psychoprophylaxis.* In 1967, physiotherapist Elisabeth Bing brought out her wonderful practical manual *Six Practical Lessons For An Easier Childbirth.* I read the book and found it invaluable in structuring the coach's role. Results were reassuring: couples became closely involved with each other during preparation, and the intensity of their relationship seemed to deepen as birth approached. Moreover, the men were delighted with the opportunity to help and participate.

I was surprised at the results. Although the Lamaze Method does not deny the existence of some physical pain in childbirth, promoting rather, "childbirth without suffering", a large number of the women did in fact report "childbirth without pain." The term "Prepared Childbirth" is now loosely used to include a number of "methods" — most based on the same principles. Lamaze classes are generally defined as preparation of the couple as a unit, using Pavlovian conditioning techniques with the father (or friend) as coach.

"Modified Lamaze" is often advertised, implying that the basic neuromuscular control and breathing techniques are used — usually with less emphasis on the conditioned reflex and possibly without a coach — although the woman may be encouraged to practice at home with her partner.

In addition to almost six hundred Lamaze courses given in the United States and a rapidly growing number in Canada, British childbirth educators, Sheila Kitzinger, author of *The Experience Of Childbirth,* and Erna Wright, author of *The New Childbirth,* have added personal modifications to basic psychoprophylaxis and have a wide following of classes which state their techniques as "Erna Wright" or "Kitzinger" approach.

Generally speaking, every childbirth educator modifies a basic method; indeed every couple modifies and adds to it in labor.

Is Lamaze "Natural"?

I have taken part in many discussions of what "Natural Childbirth" is and whether Lamaze childbirth is "natural" or otherwise. Read's definition of natural childbirth as basically unobstructed physically or mentally is a good one but I'm not sure that psychoprophylaxis fills that definition. I tend to view Lamaze techniques as "artificial" in many ways although extremely effective. It seems to me that with Lamaze childbirth we're spending a lot of effort learning a series of precise techniques which would perhaps come "naturally" (relaxation and breathing) given different cultural attitudes.

The word "natural" for many women implies primitive or "unattended". But unattended birth is not always easy and without suffering. It is impossible to write of "natural" without taking into account cultural norms and attitudes. Certainly I see even the prepared and non-medicated hospital births as "unnatural" purely from Read's definition of "unobstructed" — although they may be relatively pain-free and extremely satisfying.

Frederick Leboyer: Birth Without Violence

The childbirth education movement began with the improvement of the mother's lot, then came concern for the father. In his 1975 book, *Birth Without Violence,* French obstetrician Frederick Leboyer challenges traditional treatment of the newborn infant, believing it to be needlessly violent.

Leboyer has attended 10,000 births and observes that the bright lights of delivery, immediate clamping of the cord, forcing the lungs into sudden action, the noise and frequent rough handling, the sudden extension of the baby's spine and the dramatic change from a dark, quiet and supported environment to the exact opposite make the birth transition dramatic and traumatic. To this violent transition he ascribes what we have come to regard as newborn norms: the contorted face, screams, wildly thrashing limbs. He concludes that the child is in agony — indeed he compares the "mask of agony" to the expression of Vietnamese children burned by napalm.

Based on the assumption that the newborn is a person, he has developed a delivery approach to minimize trauma. Lights are dimmed; the room is quiet; the cord is allowed to finish pulsating with blood carried over from the placenta — giving the baby a dual oxygen supply as the lungs gradually begin to expand. The child is placed first in a fetal position, the skin gently massaged. Only after the child starts to explore the environment with arms and legs is the spine extended. A warm bath allows him or her to relax once more, quietly, in weightlessness.

"Depending on whether the transition of birth occurs slowly, gently — or brutally — in panic and terror — birth becomes a peaceful awakening . . . or a tragic one," he says.

Just as the prepared childbirth movement and the participation of the father were at first scorned as "fads", Leboyer's principles are at present under fire. In some areas they are gradually being incorporated into deliveries and I believe that the next few years will see far gentler management of newborns.

Up the Revolution

Until the early nineteen-seventies, it was far from routine for the father to attend delivery; only a handful of doctors in the entire city of Montreal allowed it. More and more fathers from my classes began to feel that the natural place for them was beside their partner at the birth of their child. More and more became insistent that they attend the birth.

On one occasion Dr. M. met me in the hall and snapped, "If you suggest to your men that they ask to be present at delivery, I'll stop sending women to classes." He did — for two years. Then a staff member and patient of his became pregnant, attended classes against Dr. M's advice, and demanded that her husband be present. He was. I watched as he supported his wife's shoulders as she pushed their ten-pound son into the world. It was a beautiful moment and Dr. M. was convinced. He now admits all prepared fathers to delivery. This negative attitude on the part of obstetricians was a tough nut to crack. But it is a battle that can and has been won in hospitals all over North America.

In 1970, my childbirth classes were the only ones for *couples* in the city — along with being the only hospital evening classes. Couples delivering elsewhere began to flock to the Booth for classes. Overcrowding became a problem. I was sole charge physiotherapist with no assistance and I was teaching two and three nights a week. Hospital administration passed the rule that only couples delivering at the Booth could attend classes there. Several doctors suggested that I start private classes to accommodate their patients delivering elsewhere. I did, and before long the phone calls from disgruntled parents began. They told tales of staff who were not only unfamiliar with Prepared Childbirth but unsupportive and in some cases hostile; of medication being given with no explanation of why it was being administered; and of fathers who were discouraged by staff in their role of coach.

In order to see firsthand the problems faced by couples in delivery, I began to accompany clients through labor and delivery at most of the English-speaking hospitals in Montreal. At hospitals where the father was not permitted to attend, I would coach his partner through the birth. Where the father was allowed, I would stand by as an observer. Despite the reports I had been given, I discovered that the staff were not all hostile. Many were merely uninformed about couple-oriented childbirth. After seeing what we were doing, and listening to an explanation, they became extremely supportive.

However, other staff members still viewed childbirth as an illness rather than a normal physical function, and could not accept the lay person's choice in techniques and method.Furthermore, the active role of the couple and the decision-making called for in Prepared Childbirth upset and irritated them. The couples' demands to be considered as individuals were viewed as a potential threat to the smooth-running hospital machinery.

"Here comes another one of *those*," staff members would sigh as yet another couple arrived bearing the tell-tale "Lamaze Goody-Bag." (Inside would be, among other things: a rolling pin and talcum powder for back rubs; lollipops, to relieve the woman's dry mouth; and a washcloth, to cool the forehead.) In one instance I received a curt memo from an irate head nurse telling me that my couples' practice of sticking a small photo on the wall as a focal point (to help the wife's concentration) would cause the walls to peel.

By 1972, the telephone calls from couples jangled day and night. My husband, David, was also drawn into the controversy. We became angry. Couples were being cheated of what we knew could be a marvelously close, shared experience — and for no good reason. We sent a letter to obstetrical staff at major hospitals and to anyone in the community concerned with obstetrics, inviting them to a meeting at our house. The purpose: to form an organization which would combine the efforts of the lay and medical community to promote Prepared Childbirth, improve communication, and upgrade existing services. Sixteen professionals and four couples who had experienced PC were present. We formed the Montreal Childbirth Education Association. The group was not designed to give classes — as we felt the problem went deeper than that — but as a lobbying group to work closely with Montreal hospitals. As a result of the MCEA's public meetings, many couples began to grow excited about PC and ask their doctors for the type of childbirth experience they chose.

In the spring of 1972, I became pregnant, and David and I found ourselves with a real vested interest in "How to Get the Childbirth You Want." I believe that it's normal for a woman to fear the unknown experience of childbirth. At any rate, despite all my training, I was somewhat apprehensive — although possibly less so than most women. Because I had extremely strong feelings about the childbirth I wanted, I chose my doctor carefully. David and I wanted to be together throughout. I did not want stirrups used, did not want an episiotomy if it was at all avoidable, and I wanted to nurse my child immediately after birth.

I was teaching at one of the most enlightened and "family-centered" hospitals in North America, but nevertheless I knew that my requests were slightly contrary to hospital routines. Because I wanted to be sure that I had a doctor who would give us as much choice as possible, I asked one with a reputation of being "liberal" whether he would go along with all of our requests. He said he would — but I was worried that he would not make it in time for delivery; his colleagues had slightly different attitudes and not all of them evaluated the need for episiotomy on an individual basis.

Fortunately everything went according to plan: no shave, no enema, no stirrups, no episiotomy (I had a small tear which gave me no discomfort later) and I nursed immediately afterwards. Our final, admittedly outrageous request in this small fundamentalist hospital was to celebrate Tilke's birth with a bottle of champagne. We did, but the head nurse, a good friend, made sure that nobody came anywhere near the delivery room while we toasted Tilke's arrival from regulation paper cups.

I realized later that even though I was on staff, and knew all of the medical personnel, I had been anxious about whether I would get what I wanted. What hope then, for the average couple without much knowledge of what is available and how to get it? David and I had experienced a perfect birth. Now we were doubly motivated to help other couples. But in summer of 1973, the roof fell in. The Quebec government decided to close the Catherine Booth Hospital in a move to centralize maternity care — and the MCEA found itself in the middle of a desperate battle. Thousands of couples protested the closing of the only hospital in the city in which fathers were not only routinely prepared for birth — but where they were *welcomed* during labor and delivery. Nearly all of the Booth's doctors had become enthusiastic about the benefits of the father in the delivery room. Staff were familiar with Prepared Childbirth and supportive of couples using it. Delivery procedures were flexible; families were separated as little as possible during the hospital stay; mothers and babies were given every opportunity to be together in an unhurried way.

A barrage of letters hit the press. Staff at other hospitals were amazed at the intensity of feeling. We organized a public demonstration. Singing a song of protest to the Minister of Health, Claude Castonguay ("Hey, hey, Castonguay, we want babies *our* way . . .") about five hundred men, women and children marched downtown to protest the loss of this family-centered maternity hospital.

We lost. The Catherine Booth Hospital was turned into a rehabilitation hospital. But its closure acted as a catalyst to change obstetrical practices throughout the city. As guests on several hot-line radio and TV shows, David and I were swamped with calls from couples who had enjoyed positive birth experiences and were prepared to fight for the rights of other couples — and from couples who had unhappy memories of childbirth and were not going to risk a repeat for their second child. As a result of community pressure, Montreal hospitals liberalized their policies. The issue of the father in the delivery room has been won almost completely, and classes for couples have mushroomed all over town.

I have related the story of the MCEA's struggle for Prepared Childbirth because I believed it is typical of events

in many North American communities today. The issue of the
father in the delivery room is perhaps the most obvious element of a revolution — in which so-called "radical" medical
and lay people are pitted against the more conservative
members of the medical community. The few radical doctors
who are willing to try the new method find themselves in the
forefront of a revolution as more and more couples look for a
doctor who is willing to give them what they want. Eventually, the momentum becomes so great that all but a few conservative doctors give in. (In one Montreal hospital, the chief of
obstetrics swore that no husband would gain admittance to
the delivery room — but many doctors sneaked the husbands
in, if the Chief was off-duty. After the Booth was closed, the
Chief was forced to change his policy — or risk losing hundreds of couples to more liberal hospitals.)

In nearly every delivery room in North America today, the
fight for father's rights in childbirth has been won, with
regard to vaginal birth. But the same battle which was fought
in the late '60s and '70s is being repeated today in another
area — the Caesarean birth. The premise for a father's presence at the birth of his child does not change — to share the
birth of his child and support his partner at this time. Currently thousands of parents share feelings of profound disap-
pointment when, because the birth has been by Caesarean section the father was not permitted to attend. Those hospitals
which offer genuine family-directed care are not only including, but welcoming prepared fathers to sit by their partner's
head at a Caesarean birth (see Chapter 8).

Furthermore, simply allowing fathers to attend does not
ensure a truly effective Lamaze birth. The joy of the shared
childbirth may be present — but it's often masked by anesthesia, or in some cases, the centuries-old suffering of women
giving birth.

As Fernand Lamaze pointed out, the pain of childbirth can
be totally eliminated for many women — but only if all
members of the medical staff understand and support his
method. While I visited Lamaze's old stomping ground,

Château Belvedere, I spoke to a number of women who had just given birth. All stressed the absence of pain — along with the hard work involved on the part of the woman, coach and staff. Director Dr. Pierre Vellay, who assisted Dr. Lamaze at the first psychoprophylactic birth in the West, in Paris on March 8, 1953, told me, "Even the person who admits the couple must be familiar with the method, or she may cause deconditioning by negative cues."

That statement became my guiding light when I was asked to set up a birth room and a related staff training program at a large Montreal hospital. In this living room-bedroom for prepared parents, birth occurs without interruption, intervention or drugs, backed by the full support of a prepared staff. The elimination of anxiety-producing procedures in this home-like setting dramatically back-up Dr. Vellay's observations about pain in childbirth. In Chapter 12 I shall discuss the hospital birth room in detail.

Yet even under far-from-perfect hospital conditions, parents in my classes are managing to actively control their birth experiences and bypass unnecessary routines by using my Ultra-Prepared Childbirth techniques to work within the system, and get what they want.

In the following chapters I'll discuss the rights which I believe must be given each couple in order to make birth as easy, healthy and fulfilling as possible. Furthermore, I'll outline my "UPC" techniques which you can use to work with medical staff — and thereby acquire these rights.

5 The right to a supportive doctor

I visited my doctor for my regular prenatal checkup . . . I told him that my husband and I were participating in Prepared Childbirth classes. His only comment was "Oh."

I asked if, providing there were no complications, my husband could accompany me through delivery. He told me that provided the staff weren't too busy, depending on who the doctor on call was and if there were no complications, it might be possible. Then he added, "That's the last thing in the world we really want — the father in the delivery room."

He told me I would be having an epidural anesthetic as he didn't want me "screaming and yelling". This is my second pregnancy. Our first child was born almost four years ago in England, with the help of Prepared Childbirth. It was a wonderful and thrilling experience which I will never forget, and without medication. I was awake, I saw my baby being born, I heard him cry.

Then the doctor said that my second baby would probably be induced so he could guarantee to deliver me. In other words, it would be more convenient for him! My first child was induced because it was medically necessary and I wanted the pleasure of having my second child arrive in his or her own good time.

I asked if I would be allowed to breastfeed on the delivery table. He told me this was not allowed. I told him I had nursed my first child for nine months and he told me that three months was long enough and nine months far too long. As for episiotomy? He said it would be done routinely. I was surprised as I had not had episiotomy for my first child and had assumed that this time the need for episiotomy would be decided on at delivery.

My last question and his reply upset me more than anything else. I asked whether my hands would be strapped. He answered, "Yes, because I don't want your hands flopping around and getting in the way when your baby is being born." My immediate reaction was claustrophobia coupled with a surge of anger, welling up in my chest like a tight knot. I believe in co-operating with the doctor, but I won't permit my hands to be strapped down. . . I am not some sort of wild animal that has to be pinned down; I am a woman about to undergo a natural and beautiful experience, and I should be allowed to have the dignity it deserves.

I have no objection whatsoever to having medication or being induced provided that it is genuinely needed. But during the entire conversation it was impressed upon me that I really had no say in the way my child was to be born.

—Norma Down.

Norma Down changed doctors and gave birth to a beautiful daughter, my second godchild, in early 1974. I watched as she and her husband participated in the birth with the dignity they had wanted.

Had she not changed doctors she would have settled for a less gratifying childbirth. Doctor "shopping" is becoming more and more common today, as more and more couples refuse to compromise with a doctor who will not allow them reasonable choice in the childbirth experience. Each week I receive phone calls from women unhappy with their doctors, asking for names of more flexible and supportive doctors. Helen's comment is typical, "He just seems indifferent and he makes me feel a nuisance for taking up his time. It's not even anything I can put my finger on. He says he allows the father to be there, but he shows no interest in the preparation Jim and I are taking, never asks how the classes are going and just seems to want me out of his office as soon as possible."

Contrast this attitude with that of Dr. Pierre Vellay. In Paris, I watched him at work in his office, attending births and making post-partum visits. Above all, he believes in the concept that woman controls her own body during birth and is the central figure — that *she delivers her baby!*

World famous proponent of the psychoprophylactic method (PPM), he maintains that the doctor must take an active part in the couple's education. In his office, no woman is rushed. As I sat in the waiting room there were never more than two, sometimes three women. Each woman was with him fifteen to twenty minutes; I couldn't help contrasting his office with the waiting rooms of North American doctors, where sometimes as many as fifteen women wait for as long as an hour, maybe longer for a five minute "visit."

In Dr. Vellay's waiting room is a blackboard with the times of the course for *Accouchement Sans Douleur* (Painless Childbirth). He teaches one class for couples in early pregnancy, explaining the normal anatomy and physiology of pregnancy and labor, emotions and attitudes of man and woman and discusses the bad effects of "psychological pollution." Psychoprophylactic techniques are taught by a physiotherapist or nurse-midwife, and Dr. Vellay gives one session on labor and delivery as part of this series. "In order for childbirth to be really painless, everyone must be very positive. If even the man at the admitting desk says to the woman 'Oh, you have a pain' — bang, the harm is done. But if he says, 'You are having a contraction, is it difficult, no? — come this way,' then the woman does not feel pain."

During my week in Paris and on his subsequent visit to Montreal, during which he spoke to the Montreal CEA, I learned his ideas on every aspect of childbirth.

On labor and delivery: "Childbirth is like mountain climbing, a lot of difficult work to get to the top of the mountain, but exhilaration when your reach the top." On induction: "I do not induce first babies. I do not believe it is safe."

On drugs in labor: "I occasionally use them when it is necessary. More than 80% of the time it is not necessary . . . I am against the epidural for normal birth because the woman is numb from the waist down."

On fathers: "The father is a very important part of the birth: it is his child as well as the woman's."

On forceps: "I was at the Mayo Clinic in the United States once. I was shown into a delivery room. There were so many people. There was the chief obstetrician, and the assistant obstetrician and one or two interns. There was the head anesthetist and an assistant anesthetist and several nurses. In the center was something — he, she? I could not say — it was completely covered. I asked what was happening and I was told that this was a normal birth. The head obstetrician was about to use forceps and I asked what the complication was and I was told, no complication. Why is she not pushing? Because she cannot push so we are using forceps. Just then we turned around to the woman. While I had been asking all the questions, she had pushed the baby out!"

On episiotomy: "I do episiotomy if it is necessary. Maybe it is necessary in about 40-45% of women. But if there is room and the woman is pushing well, the perineum adjusts itself and there will be no tear."

On mother-baby separation: "I give the baby to its mother right away. It is her child. No, we do not separate the two. An hour or so after birth the woman walks down the hall with her baby to her room. Birth is not an illness, why should the woman be confined to her bed?"

On group practice. "I attend all my own patients. Yes, that means seven days a week, twenty four hours a day on call."

On negative doctors: "If the doctor is negative how can you have painless childbirth?"

On opposition to psychoprophylaxis. "There are two reasons why this has not caught on rapidly. One is that American women are conditioned to believe that drugs are necessary for labor. The other is that doctors are not supportive. The doctor must work hard with this method. He must take time to explain. He must be there to assist with the process."

Currently, doctors learn about Prepared Childbirth mostly from observing prepared couples give birth. I have organized talks and informal discussions between medical students and prepared couples. The students receive the information with enthusiasm and these become the supportive doctors. A group of doctors attended Dr. Vellay's talk at McGill University. Afterwards one came up and said, "We've got to get this at our hospital."

Vellay says, "In France we have the same problems with doctors. PPM is still not taught in medical schools, only to midwives. I was in Rome last September. One doctor was opposed to PPM. After two days of listening to me he said, 'Yes, every woman should have a psychoprophylactic birth.' He is including three pages on PPM in his new medical textbook."

Believe it or not, three pages of Prepared Childbirth techniques in a 500-page textbook is a gigantic step forward. Medical schools today rarely teach the principles of prepared childbirth. One standard textbook, McLennan and Sandberg's *Synopsis of Obstetrics* spends about twelve lines on the subject: "The term 'natural childbirth' is used to describe a system of treating and educating the pregnant woman, with a view to eliminating her fears of pregnancy, and helping her to accept and bear the discomfort of delivery. . . . "

In the entire book — and in most obstetrical texts — the father is not mentioned once! So perhaps it is not surprising that the average doctor is not only not familiar with but indifferent to or actively non-supportive of P.C. Susan's is all too typical: "I asked my doctor what he thought of Prepared Childbirth, and he said, 'Most women can't do it.' What did he mean?"

Medical training deals in pathology — the study of sick people — and obstetrics is no exception. Doris Haire quotes one European professor as saying, "Since all the physician can really do to affect the course of childbirth for the 95% of mothers who are capable of giving birth without complication is to offer the mother pharmacological relief from discomfort and to perform an episiotomy, there is probably an unconscious tendency to see these practices as indispensable."

In all likelihood, the North American obstetrician has never watched a normal, non-medicated birth in his training, nor viewed birth without episiotomy. It is not surprising that he is not skilled in the techniques necessary to prevent episiotomy. "You'd think the resident had never seen a non-medicated birth," Andrea laughed, "He watched us and he kept saying, 'It's amazing'. He went off and brought some students in."

Jane agrees, "The doctor came in when I was doing my accelerated breathing and Brian was rubbing my back. He asked what we were doing, and I told him the Lamaze Method. He looked blank."

Unfortunately, the lack of familiarity with Prepared Childbirth can often demoralize the couple. Marcie says:

> *I told the resident that I was using psychoprophylaxis and he quipped, "Is that some sort of birth control?" That wasn't funny to me. I began to wonder if we were doing something wrong, because I expected him to have heard of it. He came in later and Al told him he thought this was transition. The doctor just looked him over and said, "I don't understand all those big words. What's transition?"*

Many well-meaning doctors fail to support Prepared Childbirth — through ignorance rather than conviction. Some time ago I participated in a panel discussion of "Women And Their Bodies" for a large group of medical students. Also present was the chief of a large obstetrical unit in the city. He talked about respecting the wishes of the woman in labor and added, "I don't believe in letting a woman suffer. I believe we should give her something for pain as early as possible, before it really gets bad. I like to give women an epidural at about four centimeters." He meant well. He is a kind and gentle doctor, but his attitude of protectivism is one which many doctors share. Many doctors cannot grasp the idea that a large number of women would rather experience body sensations and participate rather than be "spared".

At this conference I discussed what women and their partners are looking for with Prepared Childbirth: the right to be informed about methods of working with labor; and the right to have some say in the decision-making — to give "informed consent". One woman student stood up and said that that sort of choice was only for a "certain kind of highly educated woman". She added that most women want to be "looked after" and did not want to make choices. I know this notion is untrue. Yes, one can generalize that more "highly educated women" are referred to, or ask for childbirth preparation classes. But they ask to share the decision-making because they know the choices. In other countries, Prepared Childbirth is not reserved for the highly educated; certainly, my classes have included couples from every level of education and income. Education has little to do with the couple's wish to experience birth in their own way. I have found that few women express any desire just to be "taken care of" or as one pharmaceutical advertisement puts it in a promotion for a childbirth medication, to be "babied through childbirth". The majority prefer to inform themselves and take an active part in their birth. A woman about to give birth is on the verge of perhaps the most responsible and adult role of a lifetime — that of being a parent. To baby her through childbirth is a curious beginning for this role.

The Supportive Doctor

"I'm not too happy with my obstetrician," Susan told me over the phone:

> *I have a hemorrhoid and when I went to him yester-*
> *day I told him and he said, "Well, that's woman's lot*
> *and there's nothing Women's Lib can do about it." It*
> *might have been a joke, but I didn't like the way he*
> *sounded — almost pleased. I asked him if it would get*
> *better after the baby was born and he said, "Probably*
> *not." I asked if I could have rooming-in and he just sort*
> *of shrugged and said, "I suppose if that's what you*
> *want." I want to make an appointment to see another*
> *doctor but I'm wondering if there's something wrong*
> *with me.*

There was nothing "wrong" with Susan. She is one of many women who change doctors. Many of the women in my classes have changed doctors, some in very late pregnancy. "I switched two weeks before my baby's birth," Joan R. says. "All through my pregnancy my doctor had been vague about whether Morrie could be there at the birth, and I mustered enough courage to ask her point-blank, can he or can't he? She gave me a lot of maybe's. We really wanted to be together so we phoned another doctor and he was very understanding and we switched. We're really glad we did. Our only regret was that we didn't switch earlier."

What can you realistically expect from a supportive doctor? In addition to good routine prenatal health care the following are components of a truly supportive doctor:

- willingness to answer your questions accurately.
- a brief discussion of drugs and pregnancy, information about any drugs he prescribes for you — their use and possible side effects.
- nutritional information or referral for nutritional counselling at a first check-up.
- referral to childbirth preparation classes, preferably

couple-oriented.
- accurate information about any tests or diagnostic procedures that he deems necessary.
- a supportive attitude to the father's role.
- a brief discussion of breastfeeding and support for the woman's decision to breastfeed.
- a reasonable choice in the way your labor and childbirth are to be conducted.

1. Answering your questions

"Don't worry, I'll take care of you," is not very reassuring for the woman who wishes to discuss aspects of pregnancy and labor. The supportive doctor will make it his business to promote psychological as well as physical well-being in pregnancy, giving the woman opportunity to ask about her concerns. "I'm always too nervous to ask questions," Lucy says, "And my doctor's rather intimidating. I just don't have the nerve." Possibly that doctor discourages question-asking. Most doctors are busy, but you should not be made to feel so rushed that you are hesitant to ask questions.

2. Drugs and Nutrition

"My doctor told me not to drink milk because I would gain too much weight," says Lucy. "He didn't explain exactly why and he didn't go over any foods that would make up for milk. I asked what I should be eating and he said, "A well balanced diet and as little of it as possible."

Unfortunately, Lucy's doctor is typical of the majority of obstetricians in his vague approach to nutrition. Any veterinarian can tell you that maternal nutrition is an important element of animal husbandry; similarly, good human prenatal care includes detailed nutrition information.

At the first visit a really aware doctor will mention the possible danger of drugs in pregnancy and stress the importance of good nutrition.

If he feels that any medications are necessary, he should outline any possible side effects, giving you some say in the decision to take medication.

An aware doctor gives adequate nutritional information, either in the office or by printed material, or better yet, refers you to a dietitian or classes which include a session with a dietitian. He/she makes it his/her business to know that you are getting nutritional information as soon as possible in pregnancy.

3. Childbirth Education Classes

My doctor didn't see the point in classes and so I didn't think they were necessary. I'd heard of prenatal classes, of course and had friends who'd taken them, but it was the doctor who influenced me in my decision. I was nervous about the birth and wanted to ask all sorts of questions, but the doctor assured me that I would have an epidural and wouldn't have any pain. During the delivery, I hadn't a clue what was happening and kept asking for an epidural. They said it was too early, but I was in pain. My doctor didn't arrive until just before delivery — a lot he knew about whether I'd have pain or not! As it turned out, the epidural didn't take. My husband left the delivery room because he couldn't stand it. I really wished I'd taken those classes.

—Susan D.

Her experience is far from uncommon. But every woman has, I believe, the right to the necessary classes and information to prepare herself physically and psychologically to cope with the sensations of labor with a minimum of drugs. Unfortunately, even if classes are available, many women will share Susan's experience — most doctors don't stress the need to attend. Classes provide information on physical well-being in pregnancy, and teach exercises which will maintain the tone of muscles under stress in pregnancy and birth. Classes help make pregnancy more comfortable. Doctors who do not stress the need for these are denying a woman comfort not only in labor but in the months leading up to it.

The supportive doctor will mention the value of the father attending classes and will give the woman a list of classes which are couple-oriented. If there is only one class in town for couples, a supportive doctor will know about it.

4. Information About Tests

"I'm in the hospital and I don't know when I'm going to be let out," said Hester W., nearly in tears. She was phoning four weeks before her expected due date to ask about some tests which her doctor deemed necessary. "My doctor just said the baby is small and they want to do some tests. I asked him what tests and how long I'd have to stay in hospital and he just sounded irritable, 'I have a cold and I'm leaving on vacation tomorrow. Another doctor will see you,' was all he said. I've had all sorts of tests but nobody has told me what they're for. I just want to know what's happening."

Her husband Simon came alone to their class the following evening. He was anxious and uneasy about the health of the baby — angry too, that nobody was putting Hester's mind at rest. As it turned out, the tests had been done to determine the function of the placenta, or the possibility of "fetal malnutrition". Hester was sent home three days later but she was nervous and depressed for the three weeks before she gave birth — to a healthy, normal baby. "It wasn't the facts which upset us so much, it was not being told anything and imagining the worst," she said and Simon agreed. "We're not children. It's our child and we have a right to know his or her condition and the reason for any tests which need to be done."

This is not an isolated example. Frequently couples phone to ask me about tests in which the doctor has not explained either reasons or procedure. In case of uncertainty, parents naturally assume the worst. They don't ask the doctor "why?" because they are either too intimidated or too hurried.

The supportive doctor makes it his/her business to give accurate information about any tests or high-risk procedures he/she feels are necessary and also gives a realistic picture of the prognosis to his knowledge. Hundreds of couples in my classes have told me that in the case of real complications, they would prefer honesty and reassurance to worry and uncertainty. "If something is wrong we'd like to know and be given a chance to make a well-informed decision," Jim says, and most prospective parents would agree.

5. Support For the Father's Role

The supportive doctor knows that the father's participation in pregnancy and birth is vital to the growth of the couple's relationship. "Our doctor is marvelous," Ric says, "I feel included in the pregnancy. He lets me listen to the baby's heartbeat and explains things to both of us. He's pleased that I'm attending classes with Angie. He assumes that I'll want to participate in the whole thing." This doctor not only includes, but welcomes the father in every phase of the experience. He's supportive.

6. Support With Breastfeeding

All too often, the obstetrician grievously neglects discussion of breastfeeding — a normal part of the childbirth process — possibly because he concentrates on prenatal care and delivery. But the supportive doctor will mention some of the benefits of breastfeeding or at least give the woman information on the subject. Should she ask about it, her doctor will be supportive and positive rather than say, "Well, don't feel bad if you can't." A truly conscientious doctor will explain how to prepare the nipples or at least ascertain whether she will receive this information at the classes to which he has referred her.

7. Reasonable Choices in Labor and Childbirth

What are reasonable choices here? I consider that the couple should be permitted to be together throughout labor and delivery, including admission procedures and "internals" if desired. The woman should be allowed — and encouraged

— to use as little medication as she thinks necessary, or none at all if possible; to choose the position in which she feels most comfortable to give birth; to avoid unnecessary episiotomy; to nurse the baby immediately after birth if she and the baby are healthy. The supportive doctor does not unduly pressure the woman into induction for his own convenience, nor use any procedure just because it is "hospital routine." He/she will give the couple opportunity to discuss the pros and cons of their preferences, where possible. If opposed to some of their requests, the doctor will take pains to explain the reasons for refusing.

If you have had a previous Caesarean birth, but wish to avoid routine repeat Caesarean, it is vitally important that you select a doctor who allows a "trial labor" (medical factors permitting). One study estimates that 37-69% of women who have had one Caesarean can safely have a vaginal birth.[1]

How to Choose Your Obstetrician

As soon as you know that you're pregnant, decide which kind of childbirth experience you want. If you've decided to opt for Prepared Childbirth rather than the traditional North American "managed birth", shop carefully for your obstetrician.

Step One: If there is a childbirth education group (CEA) in your town or city, begin here. Phone and ask for a few names of doctors who support prepared childbirth. It helps to specify "couple-oriented" if this is important to you. If there is no CEA (sometimes listed in the yellow pages under names such as "Parent Education") a branch of La Leche League should be helpful. Failing either of these, the nursing department at a community college or university or a women's centre can be a good start. If none of these approaches work, resort to friends. Make sure your friend had the sort of childbirth you would like to have. The woman who had a non-prepared, heavily medicated birth while her partner paced the halls is not usually very helpful in her recommendations.

Step Two: You're sitting at your telephone with the list of names. Where do you go from there? Admittedly, you're faced with a bit of a gamble. But you have to start somewhere. So pick one whose location is handy to your home. Or phone the one whose name you like best. (Yes, call Dr. Sweet rather than Dr. Grindle!) Ask the doctor's nurse for an appointment for yourself, and ask if your husband would be welcome. You'll learn quite a lot from her reply. The doctor you're looking for will have a nurse who is used to father participation and will take pains to make the man feel welcome. If the nurse sounds dubious about the father's presence, say the doorbell is ringing and you'll call back later! Carry on down the list.

Step Three: You're sitting in the waiting room of the obstetrician. Take this opportunity to look around. Is the waiting room packed with women who seem to be waiting eternally? This may be evidence of an overbooked, rushed doctor. Any doctor who schedules five or six women every fifteen minutes is unable to give you the type of care you'd like. This is forgivable — perhaps — if you notice that the doctor spends fifteen to twenty minutes with each woman, or if he arrives straight from a delivery. But if women seem to pass in and out of the office every two to three minutes, this may be the wrong doctor.

Step Four: You, the mother, have been checked physically; now you and your mate are in the doctor's office. Now's the time to ask questions and assess the man. Has he mentioned drugs, nutrition or classes? If so, good. If not, give him a chance. Ask him what you should be eating. If he dismisses this with "A well balanced diet . . ." be wary. If he states that he likes women to restrict weight gain under twenty pounds, be warned. Ask whether he thinks you should see a dietitian and ask whom he would recommend. If he tells you it's not necessary, pass on to your next questions. Ask about drugs, smoking — anything you're concerned about. To help you formulate some questions about a doctor's methods of practice I have included a list of questions which I compiled and mailed to Montreal obstetricians.

The Questionnaire

- Are you in solo practice or group? If group, how many are in the group? Generally speaking do you all agree on methods of practice?
- In your practice, what method of childbirth preparation do you prefer? (No method, Read, "Natural Child-birth", Lamaze, other)
- What percentage of your patients do you refer to child-birth preparation courses? (None, 25%, 50%, 75%, All)
- Which courses do you usually refer to?
- Do you refer patients for nutritional counselling?
- Are husbands welcome to a prenatal visit?
- Do you usually permit the father to attend delivery?
- What percentage (approximately) of your patients do you induce?
- If analgesia or anesthesia are needed in the management of labor, which do you most commonly use? (General anesthesia, epidural block, paracervical block, pharma-cotherapy — e.g. Demerol)
- Do you require the routine use of stirrups?
- Do you perform your own Caesareans?
- Do you use epidural (regional) anesthesia for Caesarean?
- Can fathers attend Caesarean at the hospital where you are on staff?
- Do you allow the woman to breastfeed on the delivery table immediately following birth, if mother and baby are healthy?

Using the Questionnaire

You probably won't want to hit the doctor with the entire list at the first visit; most doctors won't take kindly to such questioning. Dr. A's view is typical: "When a couple walks in here with a list of what they want I become very annoyed. Maybe that's irrational, but I figure that after all the years spent in medical training I know my job."

Part of the problem is limited time. Most couples realize that there are other women waiting outside and the doctor is keeping an eye on the clock — so leisurely discussion is usually difficult. This is perhaps why many couples have been forced to resort to short, impersonal lists.

However, you don't want to get the doctor's back up so it's a good idea to pick a few questions. Decide on your priorities. For example, "We have been reading about the Lamaze method and would like to take classes and be together during the birth. Would you recommend this?" Right away you'll find out his ideas on prepared childbirth, classes and husband participation. If he seems positive, ask him which classes he would recommend and whether most of his couples are together during birth. In conclusion you might ask how his colleagues feel about this: are they all as supportive as he seems to be about father participation?

You've now got a pretty good idea of your doctor's attitudes and you probably haven't wasted much time.

Sorting Your Information

Let's assume that the doctor is enthusiastic about classes. He seems to know a lot about it, stresses the importance of the father and appears enthusiastic about your preparing together. All the indicators are in your favor! You're fortunate. But suppose your doctor seems rushed although his answers are reassuring. For example, he's given you the name of the hospital dietitian and seems quite enlightened on weight gain. He seems rather vague about Lamaze classes, but says it's a good idea to prepare for birth, even though most women need medication. He's told you that most of "his" fathers attend the birth. You probably won't have any direct conflicts with this doctor; his colleagues all appear to think similarly and he's come right out and said yes, the father can be there. Most doctors are not very familiar with the actual techniques of Prepared Childbirth, but usually the doctor arrives just before delivery, so his lack of knowledge should not affect you too much. He's a reasonable choice, and will probably work out well.

Step Five: You've checked the childbirth classes and the hospital with which he's affiliated (see Chapters 7 and 8). You're fairly happy. At your next visit you could perhaps ask him what he thinks of: routine stirrups, routine episiotomy, breastfeeding on the delivery table and any other concerns you might have. The approach, "What do you think about . . ." seems to work best.

Birth Without Violence?

Perhaps you have read Frederick Leboyer's book, *Birth Without Violence*, and you'd like to have some of the components of this incorporated into your own birth. Realize that this method is new, and doctors tend to dismiss anything new as "faddy". If you ask about a Leboyer birth, I would suggest that you read his book carefully first.

Many of the practices Leboyer advocates require a departure from hospital routines. Take the "cord controversy" for example. (See Chapter 3). If you ask for the cord to be allowed to finish pulsating, *the shot of oxytocin given to hasten the expulsion of the placenta should not be given immediately at the time of birth — this can result in hemorrhage!* Skin-to-skin contact of mother and baby is not routine at birth, and interferes with the sterile draping which most doctors believe indispensable. The dimming of the lights may be taken as "birth in the dark"; your doctor may argue that "I need to see the condition of the baby and the perineum." (I have watched birth, Leboyer style in Holland: although there were no spotlights used and only room light for the entire birth, the baby and perineum could be seen perfectly well.) The warm bath which Leboyer advocates may be criticized because delivery rooms are air conditioned.

However, as Leboyer himself points out, his is not so much a "method" as a gentle approach to the newborn infant, which can be achieved in several ways. (For example, rather than bathing the baby, you could simply put him to your breast immediately.) Ask your doctor if he has read Leboyer's book. If not, ask him to do so.

If he is absolutely opposed, without having read the book, you're not going to get very far, but at least you know where you stand. If he has read the book and disagrees, that's a little better: he may give you some of the ingredients. For example, many of my couples' doctors are not using the spotlight on the baby's face, and are giving the baby to the mother immediately after birth with as little noise as possible and gentle handling. These simple procedures are certainly a peaceful step towards the Leboyer approach, and may result in a more relaxed and happy baby.

Remember that delivery room techniques are regarded as a "medical" question. You're getting into the "heavy" stuff — cord cutting, etc. — which the doctor views absolutely as his territory. But I have found that the doctors who are both open to change and basically couple-oriented are interested in Leboyer's work — ready to try some of it, even if they won't do the whole thing.

What About Colleagues?

Unless you're fortunate and have a family doctor or doctor in solo practice, the odds of having your own doctor for the birth will probably be one in five, sometimes one in seven. Group practice is the obstetrical norm today. From the doctor's point of view it takes much pressure off his practice. He can take weekends off, spend time with his family and not be on call twenty four hours a day — all understandable desires. But from the consumer's viewpoint, group practice may present certain problems. How do you know your doctor's colleagues think along the same lines? What if one doctor in the group has ideas totally opposite to yours — so that you're anxious at the thought of having him attend your birth? It's sometimes a problem with no easy solution, but you can take certain steps in advance to make communication easier.

Doctors, aware of the problems of the importance of continuity, have, in some areas arranged prenatal visits on a rotation basis, so that during your pregnancy you meet each

of the doctors in the group. Ask if there is any possibility of
group rotation — so that you have a chance to see the other
doctors. For a long time many of my couples made this request and as a result of much asking, rotation is becoming
more common in Montreal.

But if rotation is not the practice for your doctor, ask
about the ideas of his colleagues. Make sure that they all
support of father participation. If you have requested some
small side-stepping of routine (e.g. you would prefer not to
have stirrups or episiotomy unless they are necessary), ask
your doctor what your chances are of getting these if he is not
present. Ask if he could make a note on your chart. Suppose
it's the episiotomy question and Dr. B. in the group always
does episiotomy. Rather than risk tearing with a doctor who
is not used to managing non-episiotomy, you would probably
do well to settle for the incision. You can change groups of
course, but you might encounter the same problem. Probably
your dominant concern is father participation: if all the group
support this, you're doing well.

Doctors to Avoid

The following elements all point to a doctor who not only
will probably not encourage active participation, or couple-
oriented childbirth, but may actively oppose it.

- The doctor always calls you by your first name with no
  invitation to reciprocate. (If your doctor calls you Mavis
  feel free to call him Ted!) First name inequality often
  goes with a patronizing approach to childbirth. The
  exception might be the case of the very young woman
  and the very old doctor.
- You, the father, are made to feel uncomfortable. Sure,
  the doctor said you could come, but he only ignores you
  and makes you feel foolish for being there.
- The waiting room is always packed with pregnant
  women who wait up to an hour for each appointment.
  Once is forgivable — deliveries can happen at any time
  — but more than twice is unnecessary and inconsider-

ate. As one of my clients, accountant Bill A., pointed out after five of these long waits, "If a businessman ran his business like a doctor he'd go broke fast."

- The doctor makes you feel uncomfortable. You're too nervous or intimidated to even ask about all the things you'd like to. Perhaps you've even tried but were cut off or put down. The doctor won't give you any straight answers. In this category, Dr. A. vaguely reassures you, "Don't worry, I'll take care of you when the time comes," — and Dr. B., a "yes" person, seems to agree to whatever you suggest. But when you try to pin down either of these doctors you may end up with "Listen, don't dictate to me," which when you're in the delivery room means "I'll do things my way."

- The doctor is adamant about weight gain and threatens to put you in hospital if you gain more than twenty pounds.

- The doctor rarely or never refers couples to childbirth preparation classes believing they're "not necessary". This attitude is likely to discourage you if you're working towards Prepared Childbirth.

- If you ask, "Can we be together during birth," and the doctor hedges, be on guard. "If there are no complications . . . if I'm on . . . If the staff aren't too busy . . ." usually means "If I get the slightest opportunity you will not be together." Unless you can get a definite answer this vagueness may mean "No."

- Does the doctor induce more than 20% of clients? My MCEA survey indicates that doctors who perform inductions *for medical indications only* induce less than 10% of births — some, less than 5%. These conservative obstetricians list the following medical indications for induction: a true "late" baby (42 weeks or later, as determined *by tests*); a mature baby which seems to be small or malnourished; premature rupture of membranes; Rh sensitization of baby; previous stillbirth; diabetes or high blood pressure on the part of the mother. Unfortunately, the majority of inductions in North America don't fall into any of these categories — they're performed for convenience.

● The doctor is unwilling to discuss any choices in birth management, or is irritated if you bring up the subject. This doctor takes the attitude, "I know my job — don't interfere", and refuses to give the couple any say at all.

● You basically feel very uncomfortable with him/her even though you've tried to communicate.

Changing Your Doctor

If your doctor disagrees with you on a point you feel strongly about, and does not appear to consider modifying his/her views, you might consider looking for a new doctor. Suppose that the doctor does not allow the father to be present or is so noncommittal that it amounts to the same thing. You have several courses of action open. First, you can stick with the doctor, at least knowing where you stand. In this case, you can try to discuss the subject in more detail — an act which may help to modify the doctor's position. Or you can change doctors. If so, when phoning for an appointment with another doctor, tell the nurse what you want, "We are looking for a doctor who usually allows the father to be present? Does Dr. A?

If you change doctors, tell your first doctor politely why you are changing. Your action may influence him to change for future couples. If your doctor will not agree to some of the smaller things, (e.g. avoiding stirrups), but generally is easy to talk to and supports couple-oriented childbirth, you may decide to stick with him/her.

REMEMBER — IF YOU ARE CHANGING DOCTORS, THE SOONER THE BETTER. BUT IT IS BETTER TO CHANGE DOCTORS LATE THAN COMPROMISE YOURSELVES IN WHAT CAN BE A BEAUTIFUL, SHARED EXPERIENCE.

Working With Your Doctor

Doctors are people and should always be approached in the same way that you would like them to treat you. "I want..." is not the best opening. Remember that you are dealing with a person who has spent years obtaining specialized training. Questions verging on the medical should therefore be carefully phrased to avoid irritating him/her. The pleasant "What do you think of . . . will get you further than demands.

When I first started couple classes in Montreal in 1967, I suggested that interested fathers discuss with their partner's doctor the possibility of being present at the birth. Many doctors were opposed to allowing the father in the delivery room. But as the following couples can attest, a great number gradually changed their views — a direct result of the couples themselves.

Peggy and Doug K. were typical. Their doctor hesitated to let Doug be present; he had no experience with fathers in delivery. But they discussed their preparation, and impressed him with their calm attitude and sensible approach. He included Doug at the birth and was surprised and pleased with the couple's teamwork and the obvious benefit to Peggy of having her husband present. This doctor has become enthusiastic about father participation. Now extremely couple oriented, he recently attended a birth with one couple from my classes, in which the woman labored and delivered in the labor room — almost unheard of at that particular hospital — and assisted in a complete Leboyer birth.

Beverley S. wanted David to be with her for everything — admission, prep., internals — and David was keen on the idea. They discussed it with their doctor, who had never tried this approach before, but agreed to give it a try. Allowing the father to remain throughout labor is now routine practice for him — but still far from routine with other doctors.

Pat and Gordon B. were among the growing number of couples who want "Birth Without Violence", Leboyer style. Their doctor was not enthusiastic but was willing to listen and discuss. They asked him to read Leboyer's book. He did. He was favorably impressed with much of it, although he had medical reservations about some parts. He explained these to the couple, and they accepted his reservations. At the birth no spotlight was used and the doctor asked the staff for complete silence. The child was given to her mother immediately. This particularly gentle birth resulted in a baby which only cried for a brief period — then no more crying — and two very grateful parents, plus a satisfied doctor, who now conducts many births in a similar fashion.

Val and Serge wanted a full Leboyer birth, having read the book and discussed it at length with several doctors. The doctor was unwilling on one score only — the matter of the bath. That was solved by Serge. On birth day the couple arrived a the hospital, Serge gravely carrying a plastic baby bath as pre-arranged with the doctor. He took on the responsibility of filling the bath, making sure that the temperature was just right for the *petit bonhomme* as Parisian Serge affectionately referred to their son Michel.

Some doctors even instigate programs which will close the doctor-patient gap. Mrs. P. writes of her experience with such a doctor:

> *I took Prepared Childbirth classes in Toronto and had an excellent teacher. The only thing which I did not like was that the classes are in no way related to my doctor. I felt that I would have been more secure had my instructor delivered me. When I told my doctor, an extraordinary and compassionate man, he understood and felt a little left out, too. He didn't understand what my breathing is all about, he just knew it worked. I felt, and he now feels that he could have given me additional support in labor if he had been better acquainted with the procedure I was using.*

As a result of his experience with Mrs. P., this doctor, a family physician with a large obstetrical practice has set up classes in his own office, assisted by a nurse. And at the two hospitals where he is on staff, he is conducting a campaign to relax many of the hospital "routines."

The genuinely supportive doctor listens to couples' views and tries to be flexible. Even the unsupportive doctor can be changed — by you. That's how father participation has become generally accepted. If a woman changes her doctor after first explaining *why,* the first doctor may review his/her philosophy. If enough women leave an unsupportive doctor, he/she may decide to change.

I'm constantly watching changes in doctors' views to clients — and these changes are made by you, the consumer. All over North America, previously conservative doctors are changing their opinions about childbirth because someone had the courage to complain, and the conviction to discuss constructively how changes would help.

6 The right to a healthy baby

In industry, quality control is taken for granted, but in human production it hasn't been given a thought. That's strange, because it costs the government about one thousand dollars each year to keep a mentally retarded person in an institution. It costs us $125 to supplement a pregnant woman's diet. That can prevent almost all the damage. At birth you're programmed for life.

—Dr. Agnes Higgins,
Director of the Montreal Diet Dispensary.

One of my friends, an intern's wife, ate "junk food" throughout her pregnancy, while her husband pooh-poohed my gentle urging that she seek nutritional counselling. I looked on helpless and horrified as Maria breakfasted on toast and jam, lunched on doughnuts and—on the many occasions when her husband worked evenings—dined on sandwiches and diet colas. She was determined not to gain "too much weight" and craved only junk food. During her pregnancy she developed the "mask of pregnancy" attributed by many researchers to vitamin deficiency, and later developed toxemia, a disease of high blood pressure related to diet. Maria's son was five and a half pounds at birth. He is now three years old, has suffered from chronic diarrhea since birth, has been diagnosed as hyperactive and is now taking daily doses of the powerful and disturbing drug Ritalin, to make him bearable to live with. Even so, when Maria recently became pregnant again and expressed an interest in nutrition, her husband's comment that he would throw any "faddy" book out of the house was not entirely in jest.

Although we cannot pinpoint Maria's poor diet as the exact cause of her son's ailments, studies show conclusively that maternal nutrition is a powerful factor in the health of the unborn and newborn child. It would indeed be callous to suggest to Maria that she contributed, albeit unwittingly, to her son's problems, but when given nutrition information, most women are eager to make sure that prenatal diet is excellent. Most would rather be safe than sorry.

In this chapter I'll discuss how you can do everything in your power to give birth to a healthy baby, something that every parent naturally wants, but too often knows little about. There are two factors *which you control* that influence the health of your newborn baby: superior nutrition in pregnancy and avoidance of drugs under normal conditions.

It would seem obvious that a healthy baby is every mother's right, but too often necessary information is withheld. It is not always easy for the mother to follow a superior diet: too often she simply doesn't know what this is! Her problem is frequently compounded by doctors offhand in their approach to nutrition and casual toward drugs in pregnancy.

You, the pregnant woman, have a right to nutritional counselling and accurate information about any drug prescribed during pregnancy or labor. As well, every pregnant woman must be made aware of the potential harm caused by poor nutrition, prescription drugs and self prescribed or "over-the-counter'' remedies for minor ailments. In this area part of the responsibility rests with the consumer — you.

Some time ago I organized a meeting on nutrition in pregnancy for the Montreal Childbirth Education Association. Guest speaker was Dr. Agnes Higgins, world famous for her twenty years of research into nutrition and human production. In an adjacent auditorium, concurrent with our meeting was a seminar on learning disabilities in children. Higgins quipped, ''If they'd come over here they'd find out how many of those can be prevented!''

''When you are building a cathedral and it's time to put in the rose window, if it's not there, the building goes on, but there's a flaw. When you're building a baby and an essential amino acid is missing, the baby goes on — but there's a flaw. It may show up years later as a learning disability.'' Higgins begins her talk to parents, expectant parents and professionals. Hers is no empty claim.

She has proven clinically beyond doubt that a great percentage of birth defects and later disabilities can be prevented by good prenatal nutrition. Her studies illustrate all too well the need for prevention rather than the search for cure.

''In France, the government believes that every child has a right to good health,'' Higgins says, ''They make sure that this is so for every single child. Mothers are paid to go to regular clinic visits for prenatal care and nutritional advice. 93% attend clinic regularly from the beginning of pregnancy. They can't afford not to go. But on this continent, if a woman goes to an obstetrician that's her choice. When she goes is also left up to her. If she doesn't get nutritional counselling, it's her tough luck.''

Her opinions are dismissed by many Montreal doctors as ''food faddism'' but a number of international experts — nutritionists and social scientists as well as physicians — have independently concluded that a mother's nutrition is the most important single influence on the health of her unborn child. Among them is renowned anthropologist Ashley Montagu who wrote in his 1961 book *Life Before Birth*, ''It is by the means of the food she eats that a mother can have the most profound and lasting effect on her child's development."[1]

What The Studies Show

Several studies now prove beyond a doubt that there is a definite relationship between the weight gain of the mother during pregnancy, the birth-weight of her baby, and the incidence of newborn death and disability.

As early as 1942, Dr. J.H. Ebbs of Toronto studied the effects of nutrition on 210 pregnant women, lower income clinic patients. All patients' diets were supplemented but the amount of supplementation varied. Women in Group One were given some iron, calcium and protein in addition to their normal diets, but in quantities too small for an ideal intake. Women in Group Two were supplemented with the same nutrients but to the level of an ideal diet. Few of the women in Group Two encountered difficulties either during the pre- or the post-natal period, or during childbirth itself. Many of the women in Group One had problems in all three stages. Length of labor for the well-nourished group was half as long as labor for women in the first group. Babies of women in Group Two had no problems in the first two weeks of life; 14% of those in Group One had problems. Prematurity for Group One was 7%, for Group Two, 2%. No miscarriages, stillborns or birth defects occurred in Group Two. Illness during the first six months of life was rare among the babies of Group Two, prevalent among those of Group One.[2]

Dr. Ebbs concluded that although none of the women in either group exhibited symptoms of deficiency or malnutrition, half of the diets had proven inadequate for the unborn child. The Ebbs study disproves the prevalent theory that the child will take all it needs from the mother, and if nutrition is poor it will be apparent in the mother. Quite the reverse: the unborn child loses out when diet is insufficient for two! The findings of Ebbs agree closely with studies done in Boston, in Buffalo and Montreal.[3]

Agnes Higgins has been in charge of the Montreal Diet Dispensary for 28 years. I first heard of her work in 1972, when as a press representative for *Canadian Doctor* magazine I attended a conference of the International Childbirth Education Association in Milwaukee, Wisconsin. There I was able to interview controversial nutritionist Adelle Davis, a major force in making North Americans aware of good nutrition. I spoke to her about nutrition in pregnancy. "Why ask me when you've got the leading authority in Montreal — Agnes Higgins," she snorted.

On my return to Montreal I was able to reach Mrs. Higgins and she spoke to a large meeting of the newly formed Childbirth Education Association some months later. Her controversial statements stunned the audience. Here was a woman advocating a weight gain of about twenty five pounds — or more if the mother were underweight! At that time her advice contradicted most obstetricians: it still does — although some have modified their ideas based on the findings of the Diet Dispensary.

Agnes Higgins has worked with low income mothers for fifteen years to develop a "no-fail" method of individual nutritional counselling which produces "Blue-Ribbon Babies", weighing between seven pounds fourteen ounces and eight pounds fourteen. "The human brain develops most rapidly in the last part of pregnancy," she says. "If malnutrition occurs at this stage, cell division of the brain will be impaired. The damage is irreversible. Studies of children who died from marasmus and kwashiokor, the diseases of starvation, show that where malnutrition occurred before birth, the brain had not developed normally. Feeding the child well after it's born won't repair the damage. Everyone is fussing about school lunches — but it's too late then."

Blue-Ribbon Babies

When a woman arrives at the Montreal Diet Dispensary, a dietitian takes a medical history, a complete detailed dietary assessment ("How much peanut butter on the bread? Well, do your teeth leave marks in it?'') and makes an income assessment. If the income is below the poverty level the DD supplements the woman's diet with vitamins and a daily quart of milk, one egg and one orange.

"The important factors in planning a diet for a pregnant woman are protein intake and calorie intake," Higgins says. To have the best babies, women need between 75 and one hundred grams of protein daily. That's not all. Unless there are enough calories, that protein won't go into growth: it will be burned up as energy and that's bad." An extra 500 calories — in addition to the normal diet — is required each day by the pregnant woman. More calories are needed if the woman is underweight, under severe emotional stress, has had a previous miscarriage or stillbirth, is having a child within a year after the birth of another child, or has a combination of any of these problems.

The results of the Blue-Ribbon Baby program are impressive. Mothers who had previously given birth to several low birthweight babies with every conceivable defect gave birth for the first time to a normal infant of six pounds or more. Higgins shows a slide of a woman attending the dispensary. "She has had ten children. Only nine are living. The first seven were low birthweight babies. She came to us for the last three. These were all Blue-Ribbon Babies and are beautiful bright children. Her first child is a retarded girl who became a pregnant teenager. Her second child is a boy. He's delinquent today. The third child died at one month. The other three children are unable to perform normally in school. That's the tragedy of poor nutrition. It's the beginning of the poverty cycle."

"The first studies on effects of malnutrition were done on animals. Animals whose diet was faulty during pregnancy gave birth to babies with deformities — cleft palate, club foot and so on. The researcher who did this thought 'I've really got a lemon.' He concluded that the problems were of genetic origin. He tried another mouse, fed her an identical diet — the same results. He then tried a different, more complete diet

— normal babies. With her next pregnancy he tried a poor diet and the deformities returned. This type of research has been done with all sorts of animals and the results are always the same but doctors say, 'Oh no, that wouldn't apply to humans.' ...But we've found that it certainly does.''

In her slide presentation, Dr. Higgins shows conclusive evidence that mothers who gain less than twenty pounds have a higher incidence of babies weighing under five and a half pounds than women who gain more than twenty pounds. The more or less either side of twenty pounds, the smaller or larger the baby. Research by Eastman, Burke and others shows the increased incidence not only of neonatal mortality (death) but of neonatal morbidity (disease and deformity) in babies of less than five and a half pounds.[4] The French have come up with a guide figure, relating mortality to morbidity, says Higgins. ''It's the 2:1 rule — for every death there are two cases of defects. If the mortality rate is seventeen (per thousand babies born) as it is in Canada, there are thirty four babies with defects, per thousand live births.''

According to this rule of thumb, in the U.S., where the mortality rate is 18.5, about 37 babies with birth defects are born in every thousand live births. Research sponsored by the U.S. National Foundation's March of Dimes shows that one of every 35 children (28.5 per thousand) born in the U.S. today will eventually be diagnosed as retarded and one in every 17 children (59 per thousand) exhibits a learning disability.[5] According to Higgins, the Canadian government estimates that 15% of all Canadian children are disabled, physically or in the central nervous system. *And her research indicates that many of these congenital defects could have been prevented!*

She explains that babies weighing less than 1200 grams (5⅓ pounds) have an 80% higher chance of cerebral palsy than babies weighing over 1200 grams. ''Other defects include obvious physical defects and diseases of the central nervous system. Some don't show up until school age: those are the 'learning disabilities.' Babies between seven pounds fourteen

and eight pounds fourteen ounces have the lowest incidence
of any of these defects, so the Diet Dispensary aims for this
weight range in its "Blue-Ribbon Babies". If the diet isn't
adequate, it's the baby who suffers. We can't make babies
bigger than their genetic potential but we can help them
realize their full potential. It's always the baby who suffers —
that's Nature's way."

Higgins hastens to point out that all findings concentrate
around the median of the curve — that is, the majority. "Certainly there are four pound babies who turn into geniuses and
there are nine pound babies who aren't very bright, but we're
talking here of averages and it's in the range I mentioned that
the overall best babies occur."

But What's a Well-Balanced Diet?

"What percentage of your patients do you refer for
nutritional counselling?" I asked in my recent questionnaire
to Montreal obstetricians. I was saddened to learn that less
than 40% refer at all, and only one in four refers routinely.
So I asked a class of eight couples if their obstetricians had
stressed the importance of nutrition. Only three out of eight
doctors had even mentioned diet. One had dismissed the entire subject under "well-balanced diet". One had told the
woman not to gain more than twenty pounds. And only one
in all eight had referred his patient to the *free* Diet Dispensary.

As a result of many hours of waiting in supermarket lines, I
have become an ardent cart watcher. It's all I can do to
restrain myself from mentioning the Diet Dispensary, when I
see a pregnant woman checking out with a cart loaded with
expensive, low protein, high carbohydrate items such as
sugary breakfast cereals, frozen pies and cakes, potato chips,
hamburger helpers, reconstituted breakfast drinks, soda
pops, canned instant puddings and candy bars. Another cart-
watcher, young obstetrician André Lalonde, became a
pioneer for good nutrition in pregnancy after observing three
of his own infants. "During her first pregnancy, my wife's

doctor was very strict about weight gain," he said at a recent seminar. "She used to starve herself for a few days before visiting the doctor and then go home and stuff herself. That baby was small, and fussed and cried for the first three months, and that kind of tension can really disrupt a household. After I became interested in nutrition, the second two children were born, each weighing much more than the first. They hardly cried, and were a joy to live with."

In 1967, when I began teaching prenatal classes, it was the fashion to restrict weight gain. The most sought-after compliment in pregnancy was "Funny, you don't look pregnant!" According to one cookbook for pregnant women, written in the late sixties,

> *Excessive weight gain is detrimental to the mother and to the fetus. Overweight women have a higher incidence of toxemia, often experience increased difficulties during delivery, have decreased vigor and a diminished sense of well being. They are also less attractive before and after delivery...You can keep your figure and your husband's admiration when you have a baby in today's nutritionally enlightened society.[6]*

As a member of that so-called nutritionally enlightened society, I too was guilty of stressing the joys of restricted weight gain. Ruefully, I recall telling women that most doctors recommended a weight gain of no more than twenty pounds. That big bugbear of the sixties — toxemia — which was ascribed to "overweight" is now ascribed by nutrition authorities to inadequate protein intake, or malnutrition.

Water Pills (Diuretics)

"The frequently prescribed 'cure' for toxemia, diuretics, or 'water pills' are of no value in preventing toxemia" writes Dr. André Lalonde in "Nutrition and Maternal Health Care," 1975. "Their use should be kept for cardiac or renal disease and/or hospital treated pregnancies where swelling threatens without any other complication, careful high protein intake with complete bed rest for three or four days should restore balance to the system."[7] In a recent interview, Lalonde told me, "none of my patients gets toxemia because I make sure they all have nutritional counselling."

Many other authorities believe that diuretics cause the loss not only of "water" but of many other nutrients essential for the health of the mother and baby. Higgins says of toxemia, "When I was called into the Royal Victoria Hospital in Montreal I worked with low income clinic patients. 50% had toxemia. After my nutrition program began there were no cases, and when one did walk in, we'd get rid of it right away by feeding her properly. There are two kinds of edema (fluid retention). One is the normal fluid retention that can occur in a healthy pregnancy. The other resembles malnutrition — swelling takes the place of healthy tissue."

Dr. Tom Brewer, author of *Metabolic Toxemia of Late Pregnancy — A Disease of Malnutrition,* who like Higgins and the late Adelle Davis is opposed to diuretics in pregnancy, has worked since 1963 with low income mothers in Richmond, California. His findings agree with those of Higgins. He is the force behind Nutrition Action Group, and in the booklet put out by the group, he urges women not to take diuretics in pregnancy. He lists 28 undesirable side effects of so-called "water pills", including loss of appetite, stomach irritation, nausea, vomiting, cramps, diarrhea, jaundice, muscle spasm, headache, and skin rash.

"The above bad effects are some of those listed by the drug companies in advertising material they send to doctors or publish in medical journals," he continues. "Water pills along with low calorie, low salt diets and indifference on the part of many doctors toward pregnancy nutrition, have created a grave health hazard for thousands of women and for their unborn children." Dr. Brewer estimates that 30,000 babies each year in the United States die as a result of metabolic toxemia of late pregnancy, and thousands more live with brain damage.[8]

Despite the evidence, many doctors are still victims of the contemporary North America idea that "Skinny Is Beautiful". "What pregnant woman wants to look like a cow?" an old-school doctor asked me. But after spending each weekend for the past year observing a herd of Vermont Jerseys, I've concluded that resembling a sleek Jersey would not be all that bad!

In the Forties, a German physician alleged that: "Semi-starvation of the mother is a blessing in disguise." Many North American doctors adhere rigidly to this credo — understandable when we discover that there is no provision for nutritional instruction in the curricula of many medical schools. "Recently I gave the only lecture in nutrition in pregnancy to the McGill University medical students," Agnes Higgins told me in 1973. "The class was allotted three hours but unfortunately it was cut to two because they needed the auditorium for something else." However there are signs that the situation is changing. Higgins' supporter, Dr. André Lalonde is now teaching the first complete course on nutrition in pregnancy at McGill University's school of medicine.

"It's going to take a lot of work on those obstetricians in the business already," Lalonde told me, "Whenever we have a pregnant patient admitted with toxemia, other doctors frequently will put her on a low salt-diuretic regime. I cancel the orders and have to convince the doctor that what she needs is more protein."

For many years the medical profession has known that the normal weight gain associated with the changes of pregnancy is around twenty four pounds, which breaks down as follows:

Weight of baby	7½ pounds
Weight of placenta	1½ pounds
Weight of uterus	3½ pounds
Weight of amniotic fluid	2½ pounds
Weight of breasts	¾ pound
Weight of blood volume and extra fluid	8½ pounds
Total weight gain:	24 pounds

To restrict a woman to 18 pounds, as at least one Montreal doctor tries to do routinely, means to put the woman on a diet, losing actual body weight. "Your husband will thank me for it," he told one of my clients recently, specifying this weight gain. This doctor suggested that she eliminate milk completely from her diet because it was "fattening", and when she asked about calcium, he snorted and told her she would get as much calcium from orange juice. His patient was already suffering from extreme fatigue, nausea and daily leg cramps. Leg cramps have been related by many to inadequate intake of milk; fatigue and nausea can be usually prevented by good nutrition.

There is no magic figure for weight gain in pregnancy. Instead, there seems to be a wide range of adequate weight gains depending on medical history, body build and the underweight factor. If a woman is underweight at the beginning of pregnancy, a weight gain of as much as forty pounds may not be harmful.

Beverley gained 45 pounds in pregnancy. She had been underweight when she became pregnant and attended the Montreal Diet Dispensary throughout pregnancy:

> *My doctor told me I was putting on too much weight. He warned me about toxemia and I started being nervous about going for a checkup. I was eating everything the dietitian had advised, and I had a lot of confidence in her. But she and the doctor were telling me totally different things. I asked the Dispensary to recommend a different doctor and I changed. The new doctor went along with everything the dietitian said and encouraged me. The first doctor had threatened to put me in hospital if I gained more than twenty-five pounds, and all my friends told me I'd never lose the weight after the baby was born. But I wasn't eating any junk foods and I felt great.*
>
> *I gave birth to a nine pound baby and my labor was a breeze. I'm breastfeeding and I'm certainly not dieting.*

I'm within five pounds of my ideal weight and the baby's only two weeks old.

I saw Beverley three weeks after she wrote the above letter and she was firm and looked wonderful. She was three pounds under her ideal weight.

Eat Your Way to a Healthy Baby

1. Every day of the week you must have:
   - One quart (4 glasses) of milk. Any kind of milk will do.
   - Two eggs.
   - One or two servings of fish, liver, chicken, lean beef, lamb or pork, any kind of cheese.
   - One or two good servings of fresh, green, leafy vegetables. (A salad is an ideal way to have these.)
   - Two or three slices of whole wheat bread.
   - A piece of citrus fruit or a glass of citrus fruit juice.
   - One pat of margerine, Vitamin A enriched.

   Also include in your diet:
   - A serving of whole grain cereal.
   - A yellow or orange colored vegetable five times a week.
   - Liver once a week.
   - Whole baked potato three times a week.

(These are the guidelines given out by Dr. Tom Brewer's Nutrition Action Group and correspond with the ideas of the Montreal Diet Dispensary.)

2. At your first doctor's appointment ask him to refer you to a dietitian and ask what his ideas are on weight gain. If he restricts weight gain to under twenty pounds, you would do well to look for a doctor with more enlightened ideas on nutrition.

3. Remember: it is not healthy for you and your unborn child to go even twenty four hours without good food.

4. Do not "skip" meals ever.

5. Do not go on "crash diets". See a dietitian to assess your ideal weight and eating plan.

6. Do not take pills to reduce appetite or water pills. These

are sometimes useful in cases of cardiac or renal (heart or kidney disease) but these are exceptions which rarely occur.

7. Avoid "junk foods": commercial pies, cakes, sodas, candies, white bread, commercial cereals.

Smoking in Pregnancy

"My doctor didn't mention smoking when I went for a checkup. I was smoking more than a pack a day and he was smoking, so I guess he didn't think it too important," Janet told me. But several studies now show that women who smoke have an increased chance of giving birth to a small birth weight or premature baby (less than five and a half pounds). The inhalation of smoke by the mother interferes with the process of oxygenation to the fetus, resulting in a slowing of the growth process.

Agnes Higgins, relating the incidence of low birthweights to the degree of smoking by the mother in pregnancy does not mince words. "I tell the woman that she must stop smoking to have a healthy baby."

Dr. W.J. Simpson of San Bernadino, California, studied 7,500 women, correlating smoking habits with history of labor and health of newborns. There were fewer premature babies to non-smoking mothers than to smokers. Prematurity rate among women who smoked one to five cigarettes a day was 7 per cent. Among those who smoked sixteen to twenty per day, the rate was over 13%; between 21 and 30 cigarettes prematurity rate was 24%; over 31, 33% were premature. Her findings showed that nonsmokers had the fewest premature children. Other studies with the same findings have been done in Scandinavia, in Birmingham and London.[9] In the light of the nutritional studies mentioned earlier, anything which can be done to reduce the prematurity rate, or conversely to ensure a good birthweight, should be done. It is another tangible way in which a mother can contribute to the health of her unborn child.

In my years of teaching couples, I have had only two women who smoked heavily. Both were unable and unwilling to give it up despite the evidence against smoking. Both women had babies of under five pounds; one baby was four pounds and born with cerebral palsy; the other baby was four pounds ten and, although apparently normal today, had problems with respiration and sucking in the early weeks of life.

Drugs and Pregnancy

In 1966, in Melbourne, Australia, as I completed my physiotherapy field work, I visited a home for crippled children. I was enchanted by one particular moppet who was giggling as she learned how to bounce in a plastic bucket arrangement which would take the place of the arms and legs which she had been born without. In place of arms, her hands flapped uselessly from her shoulders.

She was a beautiful and cheerful child, seemingly unaware of her disability, but I could well imagine the heavy heart of her mother who had inadvertently, and on the advice of her well-intentioned doctor, damaged her unborn child while preventing morning sickness by taking the drug thalidomide.

The thalidomide tragedy was a world wide scandal which turned the spotlight on pregnancy drugs. In 1962, cases of children born with phocomelia, a birth defect, normally very rare, consisting of malformation or absence of the bones of arms and legs, were reported by the hundreds in Germany, Australia, Britain, Canada, Sweden, Belgium, Israel, Peru, Switzerland, Japan and Brazil. (In the United States, Dr. Frances Kelsey refused to pass it for the Food and Drug Administration and thus saved thousands of American children from tragic birth defects.) When the final count was made, in West Germany alone, 10,000 babies had been born with phocomelia.

Thalidomide was first manufactured in West Germany, sold under the name of Contergan and used widely as a sedative for a wide variety of conditions. Its sale spread rapidly to other countries. Before April 1961 Contergan had been sold without prescription and used widely as both a sedative and remedy for nausea in pregnancy. Women who took the drug in early pregnancy — when the bones of arms and legs are developing in the fetus — gave birth to children with this defect.

The thalidomide tragedy served as a costly warning: the fetus is affected by drugs taken in pregnancy, and extreme caution by the pharmaceutical companies, medical profession and general public is the only means of preventing possible damage.

"Doctors must assume that no drug taken by a pregnant woman is absolutely safe for the fetus," Dr. Peter Gillett, assistant professor of obstetrics and gynecology at McGill University, Montreal told a group of physicians at a recent course in drug therapy. "The idea that the placental barrier protects is a misconception: in many instances the placenta makes sure that the *fetus gets its share and more of drugs taken by the mother.*" He added that a physician who prescribes a drug which could harm a fetus, to a woman during her reproductive years, should warn her of possible effects to an unborn child. As well, he should find out if she has contraceptive information. Dr. Gillett believes that not to do this amounts almost to malpractice.

Doctors share a growing concern for the widespread prescription of drugs in pregnancy. Among them is Dr. Sumner Yaffe, Professor of Pediatrics, State University of New York and Children's Hospital of Buffalo, who writes, "It has been estimated that 75-85% of all therapeutic agents are not approved for use in infants, children and pregnant women because conclusive evidence of their safety and efficacy in this population is not available, but many are administered in ignorance with potential hazard to the patient."[10] The thalidomide tragedy produced marked increase in drug testing and regulations governing marketing of drugs. In 1962 at a seminar on birth defects in Ann Arbor, Michigan, specialists urged that pregnant women should avoid drugs, including even aspirin, because any drug may be potentially harmful. Studies show that the majority of pregnant women take not

only drugs prescribed by their doctors but an alarming variety
of over-the-counter remedies for everything from heartburn
to insomnia. There is no proof of their safety, despite the fact
that in spite of drug taking, the majority of women give birth
to healthy, normal children.

Ten Years of Research — Is It Enough?

In the wake of the thalidomide tragedy, Canada now has
extremely strict regulations for drug approval, including a
requirement of ten years of research on any drug before it is
marketed. In addition, Canada's Federal Health Protection
Branch of the Department of Health and Welfare sees that all
drug companies are closely supervised and inspected an-
nually, and thousands of drug products are analyzed each
year. Similarly, in 1966, the U.S. Food and Drug Administration tightened up testing and drug regulations, but
both agencies face immense problems in these areas.

All drugs are tested on experimental animals first. But not
all animals react as humans do to a given drug. The drug
thalidomide, for example did not produce any harmful side
effects in animal experiments — although later, fetal monkey
studies did show developmental dangers. Moreover there are
certain periods in fetal development when the taking of a certain drug may be harmful, while at other times it will not
produce any noticeable effect. For example, babies of women
who took thalidomide at six to eight weeks of pregnancy had
arm and leg defects — but women who took the drug later in
pregnancy had normal infants. Exact evaluation of drug-
caused birth defects in humans is difficult because it is virtually impossible to record the non-prescription drugs taken
by a woman — ointments, nasal sprays, cough medicines, etc.
are all drugs taken by millions of women each year.

After so many years of research with animals (usually more
than five years), the pharmaceutical companies generally
market the drug to doctors, for use on a limited number of
people. If there are no recorded harmful side effects in the observation group, the drug is marketed to the general public,

although many drugs will include in small print that use is contraindicated in pregnancy and infancy.

Drug testing presents problems, however, particularly in long-term effects. For example, the steroid diethylstilbestrol was used for a number of years to fatten chickens and cattle. Use of DES as animal feed was permanently banned in Canada in 1973 because of possible cancer-causing effects on humans who ate the meat. (After temporary suspension in the U.S., DES is still being used by meat and poultry producers.) Back in the 1950's, DES was widely prescribed to prevent premature labor in women. More recently, it has been used as a "morning-after" contraceptive — not always effectively, I should add. In recent years, more than one hundred teenage daughters of U.S. women who took DES have been diagnosed as having cancer of the vagina or cervix — a disease which was previously rare among young women — and thousands more have been diagnosed as having vaginal adenosis, an abnormal cell growth in the genital area.[11]

Furthermore, recent studies done on the male offspring of women given DES in pregnancy, show an alarming increase in reproductive tract abnormalities. Results from a study on rats demonstrate that 60% of male rats born to female rats given daily doses of DES for one week were sterile and 66% had lesions in the reproductive tract. In another Chicago study, ten of 42 men whose mothers were given DES in 1951-52 were found to have reproductive abnormalities. According to one estimate, sons of mothers who took DES have a 25% chance chance of sterility. But, because the men are in their early 20's, researchers do not yet have sufficient data to determine whether these men have an increased sterility rate associated with their reproductive tract abnormalities.[12]

Another problem is that a drug may be quite safe on its own — but harmful to the fetus in combination with another seemingly innocent drug or drugs. And it's impossible for researchers to test the effects of the endless permutations and combinations of prescription and non-prescription drugs which a pregnant woman may take. Several studies have been carried out to determine how many pregnant women are using how many drugs. In Texas, 156 women studied were found to consume an average of 10.3 drugs per person in the course of pregnancy. In Scotland, 97% of 911 mothers were prescribed drugs in pregnancy![13]

Dr. Sumner Yaffe quotes the Collaborative Study of the 50,000 pregnancies, done by the National Institute of Health in the United States, which reveals that 900 pharmacologic compounds were used by 50,000 women in pregnancy. Drugs used in early pregnancy include controls for "morning sickness", sedatives, bronchodilators and antihistamines. In late pregnancy, analgesics and barbiturates are frequently prescribed for headaches and functional and emotional disturbances. Other drugs frequently prescribed include diuretics, hormones, appetite suppressants, antacids, cough medicines and tranquillizers. [14]

The Tranquillizer Alert

"You could float all of the women in Canada out to sea on a raft — made of the Valium and Librium that doctors prescribe for female 'problems,' " one disgruntled medical researcher once told me. At the slightest complaint — anything from a migraine headache to nervousness or insomnia — all too often the doctor's answer is the "mild little" tranquillizer. But according to Dr. Alexander Schmidt, commissioner of the U.S. Federal Drug Administration, these drugs can cause birth defects in the fetus if taken in pregnancy. In July, 1976, Schmidt warned against the use of tranquillizers for not only pregnant women but all women of childbearing age. He cited studies which indicate a possible connection between the use of tranquillizers in early pregnancy, and infant malformations such as cleft lip. An estimated 40 drug companies market the tranquillizers under various brand names — including the popular Valium and Librium.

"These studies do not demonstrate conclusively that these drugs, taken during early pregnancy, can cause cleft lip or other birth defects," Schmidt says. "But use of these tranquillizers during pregnancy is rarely a matter of urgency." He adds that the drugs might be ordered off the shelves if manufacturers fail to warn doctors against prescribing them for women in early pregnancy or those who might become pregnant.[15] How many more so-called "safe" drugs will be proven to be potentially harmful to the fetus? The tranquillizer alert is simply one more warning that a woman should avoid all drugs in pregnancy unless she needs to take them for serious medical reasons.

Over-the-Counter Drugs

As I watch television I am urged to banish my ordinary headache with a powerful arthritis remedy, to avoid insomnia with sleeping pills, and treat my developing cold with a mind-boggling selection of drugs, each promising "more grains of pain relief" than the last. We're a drug oriented society, and the average pregnant woman is in no way immune from this. The common aspirin is taken so frequently that many people do not even consider it a drug. "I had a cramp in my groin," one woman told me, "and I mentioned to my doctor. He told me to take aspirin and it would go away!"

But even the innocent, ubiquitous aspirin may be a villain! Although much of the effect of aspirin taken in pregnancy is unknown — and many doctors believe it is safe — we do know that aspirin taken near the time of labor may interfere with the newborn's ability to clot blood. Studies have shown that the normal clotting factors were changed when the mother had taken aspirin in the week or so preceding labor. Babies born to mothers who took aspirin close to due date had more abnormal bleeding episodes. Aspirin taken close to time of birth is thought also to be a factor in newborn jaundice.[16]

Other over-the-counter remedies that you might not think of as drugs include medicated skin creams, salves, ointments, suppositories, vaginal creams and jellies, antacid preparations, laxatives, nose drops and megavitamins. Your risk in taking them may be only slight — but why take a chance?

The human fetus cannot be used as a guinea pig, and the absolute safety of any of these preparations has never been proven — particularly in combination with other drugs. The only safe approach is in avoiding all drugs completely unless they are necessary to your health or your unborn child's because of a medical condition.

Drugs in Childbirth

The rule about drugs in pregnancy — "no drug has been proven safe to the fetus" — extends also to childbirth drugs. The effects of the more popular anesthetics have been discussed in Chapter 3, but perhaps I should add that seemingly mild painkillers can also effect the fetal brain. Studies show that drugs register an effect on the electrical waves of the brain, measured by electroencephalogram (EEG) readings. Tranquillizers, sleeping pills and pain relief pills given in labor produce changes in EEG readings. Nobody knows for certain the long and short term effects of these changes. Frequently there is no noticeable effect in the newborn; occasionally there may be some drowsiness; there may be a learning disability in later life.[17]

In 1972, a Collaborative Perinatal Study was organized by the U.S. National Institute of Neurological Diseases and Stroke. 55,000 children were followed from birth to one year of age. The report, *The Women and Their Pregnancies,* compared the incidence of significant neurological damage at one year — and found a greater incidence among white children than among black. Doris Haire writes, "These findings are not so startling when one considers that, although the incidence of low birth weight, prematurity and undernutrition is decidedly greater among our black population, black patients who are more often clinic patients, traditionally receive less medication during labor and birth. (In one New York City hospital during 1970, there was twice the incidence of depressed babies among private patients as among clinic patients).[18]

Since the publication of this report, the Committee on

Drugs of the American Academy of Pediatrics has issued a warning, *"There is no drug which has been proven safe for the unborn child!"* Because it may take more than a decade to discover that a seemingly safe drug such as DES has harmful effects, members of the medical profession should approach the use of drugs in pregnancy and childbirth with the utmost caution.

Currently, pharmaceutical companies are under attack for over-promoting the use of drugs, but the fact remains that no drug company ever wrote a prescription. Drugs are a two edged sword; without them, many lives would be lost. The physician has a responsibility to read information on the drug; to avoid the use of drugs for pregnant women wherever possible, and to advise them against over-the-counter drugs and discuss any side effects possible with drugs he prescribes for a medical condition. But all too often the obstetrician treats drugs in a cavalier fashion. I recently asked eight couples attending my introductory class in early pregnancy how many of their doctors had mentioned avoiding drugs in pregnancy. Not a single doctor out of eight had so much as mentioned drugs! "My doctor put me on Valium because I was on edge," one woman told the others.

Dr. Sumner Yaffe writes, "Labels on medicines warning the doctor and his patient that the enclosed pills are 'not to be be taken during pregnancy' will do no good. The chief source of protection lies with the obstetrician filling his role as the pediatrician of the fetus. In this situation he must lead the crusade for a widespread acceptance of a sensible attitude toward drug consumption during pregnancy. This period can be rendered safe only by practising therapeutic nihilism for all women between the ages of 14 and 40 . . . Most people in our society view life as a drug deficient disease to be cured or even endured only with the aid of innumerable medications."[19]

For the safety of your unborn child, your best approach is ultra-conservative: avoid all over-the-counter drugs and discuss any drugs prescribed by your doctor for a medical condition concurrent with pregnancy very carefully. If it is considered absolutely necessary to treat such a medical condition with drugs, follow directions for drug taking exactly: the *exact dosage for the exact amount of time prescribed.* Certainly the pharmaceutical companies, the federal drug regulations boards, and the doctor must share responsibility for the use of drugs — but part of the responsibility is with you, the consumer.

Five Recommendations

Consumer's Union in the U.S. proposes five ways of reducing drug risk in pregnancy:
1. Increased understanding about drugs in pregnancy on the part of physicians and their patients.
2. International cooperation in drug testing.
3. Improved package inserts.
4. Reporting on adverse effects. (In 1951, the Canadian province of British Columbia pioneered a registry for the reporting of major birth defects. Since 1970, four other provinces have joined in a federally co-ordinated surveillance program for reporting defects detected in the first year after birth. In 1974 a similar program was launched in the United States with 1,500 hospitals participating in a Birth Defects Monitoring Program, coordinated by the Center For Disease Control.)
5. Primate tests. Testing on experimental animals usually is done on rats, mice and rabbits. But perhaps testing would be more effective on monkeys or other primates more closely related to humans. Such tests are encouraged by the Canadian and U.S. drug protection agencies, but are not required.

How to Do Everything in Your Power for a Healthy Baby

1. Follow nutrition guidelines outlined in this chapter. Choose a doctor who will not restrict weight gain to a "magic number" of pounds, e.g. "no more than twenty pounds, or else . . .!"
2. Ask your doctor for referral to a nutrition counselling ser-

vice — the nutritionist at the hospital where you are to give birth or a community nutrition centre in your area.

3. Do not smoke cigarettes or marijuana. Minimize consumption of coffee, tea and alcoholic beverages.

4. Avoid all over-the-counter drugs during pregnancy.

5. Potentially harmful effects of many drugs occur in the first weeks after a missed menstrual period, — so if you suspect pregnancy, avoid all drugs, in the broadest sense of the word (ointments, pain remedies, cold remedies etc.) and ask your doctor about possible effects of any prescription medicines you are taking. If you are trying to become pregnant, tell any doctor this, if he prescribes any medication for medical conditions.

6. If there is a medical condition which the doctor feels warrants prescription medicine, discuss any possible side effects, including those from not taking the drug, and get as much information as possible about what is prescribed for you.

7. If you and the doctor decide that medication in pregnancy is advisable, follow dosage and length of treatment to the letter. Do not skip doses and do not discontinue taking the medication too soon. For example, if the prescription tells you "take after meals for ten days," don't stop after two: the drug may not work so effectively if you stop taking it too soon. The health of your baby can be affected adversely by your not taking a necessary medication — as much in some cases as by taking unprescribed medicines.

8. If you are breastfeeding a baby, avoid drugs as you would for pregnancy: drugs are carried to the nursing baby and many are contraindicated.

9 Avoid X-rays during pregnancy unless your doctor feels they are important for diagnostic procedures. If dental X-rays are deemed necessary, make sure the dentist knows you are pregnant: a special apron which blocks the X-rays will be used in this case.

10. Minimize your need for childbirth drugs by enrolling in a childbirth preparation course to equip yourself to work with

labor.

Very few women have chronic medical conditions such as heart disease or severe diabetes, which require constant medication. For most other women, prescription medicines can be confined to use only in treatment of acute medical conditions, and are usually unnecessary in pregnancy. Over-the-counter remedies can be avoided, particularly if you follow nutritional guidelines and have superior diet. In many cases the remedy you take for a cold or other minor ailment will simply mask symptoms which will clear up nearly as quickly without any drug. By following these guidelines you are doing everything in your power to have a healthy baby.

7

The right to childbirth education

Mary L., a graduate student at a large university, became pregnant and decided that she preferred not to know too much about the process. She placed herself in the hands of her doctor whom she felt was better qualified to make decisions about delivery than she was.

Mary went into labor prematurely. She and her husband went to the hospital, where an intern and nurse diagnosed her contractions as indigestion. Her obstetrician chose not to come to the hospital to confirm the diagnosis.

She was sedated though in severe pain and sent home at 9 p.m. Her equally uninformed husband went to bed even though his wife's symptoms did not subside. At 4 a.m., while Mary thought she was passing a very stubborn bowel movement, her baby was expelled into the toilet. She quickly retrieved it. The fire department emergency squad came, clamped and cut the cord and took Mary and the baby to the hospital. The child lived but Mary was glad her daughter remained in hospital for several weeks. It was so traumatic an experience that she needed time to recuperate psychologically before the baby came home.

Meredith W. tells a very different story. She writes, "Thanks to your marvelous course, our little Beverley's birth was an absolute breeze. My memories of childbirth will now be of an elating and pleasant experience, not one of hideous pain." Meredith's first two children had been born with little preparation, in long hard, painful labors:

> *With this baby I decided that I'd do anything to improve on the last labors. I'd also had terrible pregnancies. I had a friend who had taken the course, also after two "bad" births and she had had a really good experience, so I decided to try it. My husband had been present at the first two births but hadn't prepared with me and didn't get into it at all. On this baby, he was not enthusiastic about coming to classes, but when we started practicing together he became extremely interested.*
>
> *Thanks to the exercises I had a comfortable pregnancy. The breathing worked beautifully. My other labors had been longer than twenty hours each — I'm sure that that was partly due to my tension and the medication that I kept needing. This baby was born four hours after I started labor, and weighed ten pounds.*
>
> *After I'd had the baby I couldn't believe I wasn't going to have pain. I asked the nurse for morphine. She laughed and asked why I'd want that when I'd just gone through labor not needing anything. I told her it was too good to be true and I knew the pain would start. It didn't though and next day I felt great. To his surprise — and mine —my husband can't stop talking about "our" birth!*

Meredith is one of hundreds of my female clients with unpleasant memories of a previous managed birth — who have discovered to their amazement that childbirth education can eliminate much of the fear, and thus the pain, of labor. In the case of Mary L., knowledge on the part of her and her husband would unquestionably have resulted in a fast, easy and happy hospital birth rather than a frightening, agonizing episode alone at home. Any prepared woman will recognize the signs of labor — and so will her husband. And nearly every couple given the assertiveness techniques that good childbirth education should provide (techniques which I call UPC) would have refused to leave the hospital without first having the woman examined by a staff obstetrician. Mary L.'s case is just one more instance in which the *laisser-faire* attitude of some obstetricians towards childbirth education ("Don't worry your little head about it — I'll handle everything") can result in a needlessly unhappy and painful birth. Like Meredith, about two-thirds of my clients are referred to PC classes by grateful friends rather than by obstetricians — an unfortunate statistic which I will discuss at more length in Chapter 12.

Why Childbirth Education?

Whether you are a low-risk or a high-risk case; a woman who has had several infants by other methods (i.e., so-called "natural childbirth", the epidural or other medication); a "primipara" experiencing motherhood for the first time; or the mate of any of these women — childbirth education can be of enormous benefit to you and your unborn child. Really thorough childbirth education classes will prepare you for all phases of pregnancy, labor and delivery — and the crucial postnatal period as well. Moreover, a good class should provide group interaction that will let you know that any negative feelings which you may have are completely normal. Most courses taught by qualified PC instructors have the following aims:

- to provide information about the normal process of pregnancy and to reduce or eliminate physical and emotional discomfort throughout pregnancy.
- to provide accurate nutritional information as early as possible in pregnancy.
- to provide information about breastfeeding and

preparation of the breasts during pregnancy.

- to provide an environment which allows couples to discuss feelings and attitudes to pregnancy and childbirth.
- to prepare the man and woman emotionally and psychologically for the experience of childbirth.
- to prepare the woman with physical activities which will allow her to participate in the process of labor with a minimum need for drugs.
- to prepare the father to participate in the birth of his child, and to act as "coach" should he wish to.
- to prepare the couple for the changes of parenting; provide information about the new baby and discuss possible changes in attitudes and lifestyles.
- to help prepare the man and woman for a positive, shared, growth experience throughout pregnancy, childbirth and parenting.

Since 1967, I have taught various kinds of childbirth preparation classes, including Read Method for women only; Read method including fathers at one session; Lamaze method with father as coach attending every session; Lamaze method with a woman friend as coach at each session; hospital classes; and private "Lamaze" classes in a six week series. In the last three or four years I've developed a course which begins in early pregnancy, resumes again eight weeks before birth and continues until birth, then resumes two weeks after birth for several weeks.

I have found the latter course to be the most satisfying. It allows continuity and deals with the childbearing year as a whole, rather than a fragmented set of experiences. My course is held in my home and as I outlined in Chapter 2, is divided into three sections: *Pregnancy* which begins as soon as possible in pregnancy; *Birth,* the Lamaze part of the course which commences eight weeks before due date and until birth; and *Parenting,* which commences two weeks after the birth.

Each class is two hours long and there are eight couples in a class.

Pregnancy:

This series of three sessions on consecutive weeks begins as early as possible in the pregnancy. In the introductory class, we discuss the couples' expectations from the course, the philosophy and history of childbirth education and the psychoprophylactic method. We discuss the three "issues" usually brought up when dealing with PPM (Psychoprophylactic method) — pain, medication, and father participation. I explain the anatomy and physiology of pregnancy. ("what's going on inside and what you may feel about it"), the importance of posture and basic comfort techniques for pregnancy. We look at pregnancy as a demanding but normal state — not as an illness — and discuss drugs in pregnancy.

The second class is given by a dietitian from the Montreal Diet Dispensary, who covers the importance of maternal nutrition and its effects on the developing fetus. Nutrition, lactation and infant feeding in general are discussed.

The third class begins with one hour of exercises to prevent backache, firm the abdominal and back muscles and learn control of the pelvic floor muscles. We discuss posture and daily activities in more detail. The second hour of the class deals with an introduction to breast-feeding — or the "sense and nonsense" of the subject, including the facts, attitudes and how to's.

Birth:

This part of the course begins eight weeks prior to the given due date. We cover the process of labor and how the woman will actively work with the changing sensations of labor with her partner as coach. The Lamaze principles of neuromuscular control, breathing techniques, cortical inhibition and conditioning are covered each week — with my own variations which have developed through years of coaching and instruction.

We discuss physical and emotional changes of late pregnancy, and the onset of labor. We look at the hospital environment, the "rights" which this book is about, and my 13

UPC rules, which are explained in Chapter 11. We cover the birth of the baby, the newborn and its care, the mother-baby unit and the role of the father. We discuss high-risk procedures and how to bypass them in a responsible way.

Included in this series are films of psychoprophylaxis in its French and American forms, breastfeeding and baby care. The final classes in the set are in the form of informal "drop-ins" in which couples expecting their babies soon discuss birth and parenting with new parents who come with their babies. With new fathers, my husband David discusses the finer points of coaching and the father's role in parenting, while the women discuss the immediate post partum period and breastfeeding. We rehearse different kinds of labors and discuss varying birth experiences including Caesarean section. These Drop-Ins — part rehearsal, part parent discussion — continue until birth.

Parenting:

For several years I have included this section of the course as an informal Drop-In or open discussion for new parents with their babies as well as those couples very close to — or past — the "due dates" predicted by their obstetricians. Couples drop by not only in the first few weeks after the birth, but at any time in the first year, to exchange ideas and stages of development. Sometimes older children or even grandparents attend. Couples tell me that these sessions help them enormously during the inevitable problems of the first year of parenthood.

Over the last few years these sessions have become more structured to meet parents' request for specific information, as well as group discussion. The current parenting program continues from newborn to three-months of age, with the option of drop-ins until one year. The first session is given by obstetrical nursing instructor and mother, Georgiana Kish who bathes one of the newborns (usually two to three weeks old) and discusses newborn behaviour and care, infant feeding, growth and development, baby safety in the home, as well as the emotions of new families.

Helen Cantlie, a general practitioner with a large pediatric practice, became deeply interested in tactile stimulation for the newborn, after giving birth to a child with cerebral palsy seven years ago. Helen found that through touch, and extensive use of all five senses, she was able to help her child achieve his full potential. After her third child was born recently, an easy birth using psychoprophylaxis, Helen turned her attention to the newborn and evolved a program of infant 'play' using Janine Levy's book, *Exercises For Your Baby* as a guideline. I watched as she used the techniques with her child, bringing him in to Drop-Ins frequently.

She now conducts a baby play evening as part of my Drop-In series, enabling fathers as well as mothers to participate in the play-exercises. "It's funny, but I felt a little nervous about handling Julie at first," one father told me, "I don't mean holding or changing her — that was no problem — but I wasn't sure what else to do with her. This exercise program is wonderful fun — and it gives me the parent a whole lot of things to do with the baby."

Drop-In is in many ways the most enjoyable part of the course and allows parents to keep in touch with each other. For many, these sessions are the only contact available with other parents of small babies. Many couples are new to town or simply have no friends with children of that age. It can be lonely parenting in a large city: judging from attendance at Drop-Ins, I feel that post-partum programs may well be as valuable as the birth preparation itself. My parenting program was the first of its kind in the city: today, many other childbirth educators are adding such sessions — so, with luck, an instructor in your city may hold these valuable get-togethers as part of PC classes.

Early Pregnancy Programs

I'll never forget Marilyn, a tense apprehensive woman who began classes quite late in her pregnancy, with a husband who seemed reluctant to have anything to do with the pregnancy. She had a spinal curvature, had always had it and told me that for most of her life she'd had backache. She had come to classes because the backache was so bad that it interfered with her daily activities, and told me, "I'm terrified of birth. I just know it's going to be hideously painful."

At the first class, Marilyn demoralized the entire group with her insistence that nothing would help her in labor because she know she'd never be able to take the pain. All her friends had had terrible births, she said, and she knew she would too. She was here only because her doctor had told her exercises might help her back, but she doubted his word. I was rather pessimistic about Marilyn, I confess, but we spent some time exercising and discussing good posture and daily activities. Her husband learned how to check her posture and make sure that she was doing the exercises correctly.

Several weeks later Marilyn reported a slight improvement in the backache. She and Morrie, her husband, seemed more relaxed. At the following class, four weeks after they had commenced the course, she bounced in and announced with delight that for the first time in years she was not having backache. She told the group that she had been doing the exercises faithfully; Morrie added that he had made sure that she did. Marilyn's backache did not return. Confident that the exercises had worked, she and her husband practiced the Lamaze techniques just as faithfully. I noticed that Morrie was becoming more involved with the pregnancy and with the other men in the group.

Marilyn phoned me from the hospital one hour after giving birth to a seven and a half pound boy. "The whole thing only lasted three hours," she told me excitedly. "I can honestly say that I felt no pain and you know what a coward I am." I was amazed. "Morrie was marvelous. I don't think I could have done it without him, he's so excited he can't stop talking about it to his friends." Six months after the baby was born, Marilyn still had no backache.

Early pregnancy classes are vitally important on several counts. The sooner the woman begins to exercise and become conscious of her posture the more comfortable she will be for the rest of the pregnancy. Backache, regarded by so many women as a normal part of pregnancy, can be prevented in almost every case. Other minor discomforts of pregnancy caused by pressure on other organs can be minimized by exercises and posture. Perhaps even more important is the "couple chemistry" which I've watched occur in early pregnancy classes.

Most couples attend the first class a little nervously — particularly the men, who openly admit that they are there because they want to help their partners, but are not sure of anything beyond that. As we discuss the importance of the coach's role in psychoprophylaxis, they become more at ease. For some time in our culture, man's role in childbearing experience has been a poorly defined one. Clarifying his role makes the father more confident.

We discuss normal side effects and emotional changes of pregnancy, and most couples are relieved to know that they experience similar reactions to pregnancy. "I really wasn't too enthused about being pregnant," Jennifer told a recent class. "I thought I'd made a great mistake even though we'd planned the baby. For ages it seemed I was tired and cranky and Steve thought I was just being bitchy. Now we know that this can be common we both feel a whole lot better. I think the worst thing in pregnancy is wondering whether all the things you're feeling are normal. Just knowing that they are is enough to get rid of them!"

Isabel agreed. "I've been having bad dreams. I kept dreaming that I'd given birth to a baby and there was something wrong with it each time. You don't know how relieved I was to find that other women have these dreams too."

Apart from group support, the value of nutritional information in early pregnancy cannot be overemphasized. The sooner the facts about breastfeeding are covered, the sooner the mother can make a decision on the subject and resist the "psychological pollution" of pregnancy of which Dr. Vellay speaks. (The benefits of breastfeeding are discussed in detail in Chapter 10.) Early inclusion of breastfeeding allows the couple time to read extensively (advisable in this culture which is geared to bottle feeding); gives the woman time to prepare her nipples for nursing to prevent possible soreness and time to choose a pediatrician supportive of breastfeeding. The research in this area may take some time and is best begun early!

Perhaps one of the more important areas of childbirth preparation is the information given on possible complications, high-risk procedures, diagnostic tests and Caesarean birth — all areas which cause considerable anxiety, particularly for the unprepared couple.

> *The biggest advantage of the course for us turned out to be the detailed information we were given about Caesarean birth. Janet's labor never progressed and for five or six hours she worked with strong irregular contractions as the doctor decided that he would wait to see if progress occurred. We would both have been really scared if we hadn't discussed all this in class. We knew the sort of contraction to expect from a "no progress" labor, we knew how to adjust our techniques, we knew what the staff were talking about and could co-operate fully. I think that my encouragement helped so that Janet didn't need medication prior to the Caesarean. Janet was relaxed during the whole thing and of course we were anxious but we both feel that this was minimized because of classes. In those hours of hard labor before the section, we felt we had truly shared the birth.*
>
> *Because we had discussed epidural anesthetic for section in our classes, I was able to remember to ask for it and I saw my baby as soon as he was born and heard him cry. The only improvement would have been if Scott had been with me. Next time maybe we'll get that too.*
> *— Janet and Scott B.*

Although I had difficult back labor, Don and I
worked as a team throughout and felt more exhilarated
with every passing hour. I don't think the staff at this
hospital has had much opportunity to observe prepared
couples. Consequently we received so many com-
pliments and their remarks boiled down to the two
words, "quelle différence" — what a difference pre-
natal classes make!

— *Gail and Don C.*

Howe-Elkins Procedure:
Will Breech Babies Turn?

Several years ago, Sue W., one of my women clients
worriedly informed me that her doctor had diagnosed a buttocks first presentation position ("breech") of her baby, due
in a few weeks. A breech birth is not always more complicated
than the more usual head-first delivery. But the position of a
foot or both feet first may lead the obstetrician to decide that
a Caesarean birth is safer than a difficult vaginal birth. Sue
wondered if anything could be done: her doctor had already
told her that nothing could prevent a breech birth. Quite un-
scientifically, I postulated that perhaps if the baby were given
a taste of the correct head-down position, he or she might
turn into it — rather far-fetched, but worth a try.

I suggested to Sue that she try the "knee-chest" position,
an exercise which has been in use for a long time to minimize
pressure on back and lower abdomen in pregnancy. Sue used
"knee-chest" for fairly long stretches, done at regular intervals. Within three days, the baby turned. Soon afterwards,
Sue gave birth to nine pound, five ounce Soren, in what her
doctor described as "perfect presentation"; her labor required no medication whatsoever!

But one case is very likely coincidence. Since then, 72
women whose babies were determined breech by ultrasonic
diagnosis, from the 37th week of pregnancy and on, have followed a procedure which I developed. Before 37 weeks of
pregnancy, many babies are in the breech position and the

majority will turn spontaneously. I limited my study to babies of 37 weeks and later, who are less likely to turn. 66 of these babies turned from breech to vertex and all of those were normal vaginal births: the infants weighed from six pounds fourteen ounces to ten pounds four ounces. The six babies who remained breech were all born by Caesarean. Of this second group of babies, two had a low-lying placenta; two had an unusually short umbilical cord; and one mother had an abnormally shaped uterus.

Howe-Elkins Procedure:

Fifteen minutes of the "knee-chest" position (used conventionally to relieve pressure discomforts in the lower back and abdomen during pregnancy) were repeated every two hours of waking time for five days. I checked the position carefully in classes, with particular attention to correct positioning of back, shoulders and knees. Each woman had her doctor's approval for use of the procedure.

Two-thirds of the babies who turned were diagnosed vertex (head down) after one cycle (five days) of the procedure. The remainder turned following a repetition of the five-day cycle. The women who used my procedure to turn a breech baby felt that they had nothing to lose. Gloria K., one woman using the procedure, was in hospital awaiting Caesarean when her baby turned!

If you have been told that your baby is breech, discuss the use of my procedure with your doctor. (I have not recommended the procedure in cases of a "footling" — both feet first — presentation.)

Have your doctor or childbirth educator check your position. Knees should be quite far apart, hips perpendicular to knees, back rounded and head resting comfortably on a pillow or your arms. If your arms are too far forward, your back will hollow, causing backache. Many women find the position hard on the knees when done on the floor, and prefer to do it on a bed.

Because knee-chest was so effective for breech presentation, I began to speculate on whether the incidence of "back labor" — posterior presentation in which the back of the head presses on the mother's spine — could also be prevented. I had noticed that many women who experienced back labor had mentioned an earlier diagnosis of retroverted or "back-tilted" uterus. Would the knee-chest position, a known cure for the retroverted uterus, prevent back labor as well? I began to recommend more than the usual use of the position during pregnancy, and the incidence of back labors in women in my classes started to fall.

The complete procedure is only indicated for turning breech babies. To minimize the possibility of back-labor, or for conventional use to relieve pressure in pregnancy, once or twice a day for as long as comfortable is adequate. A good childbirth educator will usually teach you the knee-chest position as a routine part of childbirth education for comfort in pregnancy.

Who Teaches Childbirth Preparation?

Traditionally, childbirth preparation has been shared by the physiotherapist and the nurse, in a hospital or clinic setting, through a community center or privately.

Hospital Classes:

The ideal hospital course is exemplified by St. Joseph's hospital in Hamilton, Ontario, developed by the former Chief of Obstetrics and Gynecology, Dr. Murray Enkin, one of the directors of the ICEA. In 1964, Dr. Enkin introduced psychoprophylaxis into the hospital and has developed a total staff involvement program for couples, given at the hospital. Classes are large and are divided into two parts. Theory is given to the whole group of about thirty couples, by a doctor, nurse, and other members of the staff. The group then divides into small groups of four or five couples with a staff group leader who supervises the actual psychoprophylactic techniques. Couples remain in the same small groups for the entire course.

Couples are shown the hospital, meet the various members

of the team and are reassured by the knowledge that when they arrive, the staff will fully support what they are doing. Dr. Enkin says, "I do not insist on shaves and enemas, and the woman can push in whatever position she feels most comfortable. High-risk procedures are used only for high risk, never normal labor. Dr. Enkin also allows the father to cut the cord. At the 1975 conference of ICEA in Hamilton, where David and I were speaking on *The Rights of The Pregnant Parent,* I discussed Leboyer's techniques with Dr. Enkin. "I find a lot of his approach creeping into my own work — avoiding the spotlight, leaving the cord for a few minutes, being gentle with the newborn. It's moving in gradually with a lot of other doctors too."

Childbirth classes in hospital can be excellent, provided they're the result of a well co-ordinated effort between various departments, as they are at St. Joseph's. There's an advantage to going to classes at the hospital where you'll give birth: you become familiar with the hospital, and with its attitudes and policies as well. But too often, hospital classes aren't well co-ordinated: what is taught in classes may have little relevance to attitudes in the case rooms. Unless there is a good in-service education program, the teaching may be inconsistent, as this is usually done on a rotation basis and shared by physiotherapy and nursing departments. I have spoken to many people teaching such courses, who have not watched their methods being used by the couples they teach! Often classes are advertised as "Lamaze", but there is no mention of the conditioned reflex, and the mate, although present, does not actively participate in preparation or coaching.

Recently a woman phone to tell me that the Lamaze Method didn't "work". I questioned her further. "I took Lamaze classes at the hospital and my husband came to every session with me, but as soon as I arrived at the hospital I forgot everything I'd learned and we both panicked." After further discussion I learned that breathing techniques had been shown in two sessions, with no mention of the conditioned response and the father sat on a chair behind his partner for the series. That was not "Lamaze".

Some months ago I was phoned by an obstetrical coordinator who told me that the hospital was thinking of "going Lamaze". She said that the doctors would not be ready to go "all the way" but she thought that maybe they could teach some of the things like "effleurage" (light abdominal massage done during a contraction). She, like many other personnel, equated the method with "natural" childbirth and was unaware of the method's basis in the conditioned response.

Some time later, she notified me that the hospital had in fact "gone Lamaze". I was pleased and thought that it would be a good beginning: she had attended Pierre Vellay's talk and seemed to have read several books. But months later I received a letter from a woman who had taken the course:

> *The nurses were excellent and their talks on prenatal development, physiology, and breastfeeding well done. The course supplied all the information tools necessary to participate in labor, but by then we'd met a couple who had taken a Lamaze course and had had a marvelous birth experience which made them enthusiastic enough to teach us what they had learned. We realized that what we were learning at the hospital was very different.*
>
> *In the classes at the hospital, because the proper application and attitude were never stressed, success would have been difficult. It is almost like dropping off some tractors and other agricultural machinery to an underdeveloped nation without any instructions. They would have the tools necessary to feed their people more efficiently, but without the proper instruction or knowledge the people would still starve.*
>
> *Conditioning was mentioned but not stressed. Very little was said about husband involvement with cues etc. Some effort was made to involve the husbands but . . .*

*the real joy of having a loving person participate equally
in the entire labor was not stressed!*

*The epidural, however, was stressed, almost as part
of the labor process, almost in fact as part of "natural"
childbirth. The nurse made it sound as though the
epidural was the most wonderful thing because it would
make the pain go away.*

*Fortunately our friends passed on the positive, en-
thusiastic approach, the detailed conditioning, the
coach's vitally important cueing and the birth of our
daughter was calm, non-medicated and a moment Ian
and I will never forget. I doubt though whether we'd
have been able to function as the team we were if we had
had only the hospital classes.*

— *Gay MacLeod*

Hospital classes can be as excellent as the ones at St.
Joseph's Hospital, Hamilton. But too often, as Ms. MacLeod
attests, hospital instructors may lack enthusiasm and proper
knowledge of techniques. For example, the hospital in which
Ms. McLeod gave birth is developing a fairly complete pro-
gram. But although the printed course outline praises
"Prepared Childbirth", one session features a talk on
"Epidural versus natural childbirth" . . .,

Hospital classes usually prepare parents for the birth norms
at that hospital. I suggest that you tour the hospital and ask
questions about alternatives available before taking the
classes. I currently direct a hospital program based on my private classes — early pregnancy, birth and parenting, with
emphasis on UPC techniques. This program requires considerable staff training and co-ordination, but has resulted in
increasing support for parents' choices — including a birth
room (see Chapter 12).

Community and Private Classes:

I've taught hospital classes, in a hospital where I divided
my time between teaching and coaching labors, and where the
staff were familiar with what couples were doing. I've also

taught classes in the community and in my own home. At time of writing I teach only privately, attending a birth or so each month and coaching occasionally. Once a month I take a group of my couples on a "hospital tour", and because of my MCEA work, I am constantly speaking with staff at most of the major hospitals. In addition, physiotherapy and nursing students sit in on many of my classes. Without this communication and hospital contact, I think my work would suffer from isolation.

One of the problems of my private course is that the couples who attend it deliver their babies at many different hospitals. So a great deal of my course consists of explaining the situation of these various hospitals. It is not enough to teach a method. The teacher must make sure that the staff will be familiar with the method couples are using. The teacher must also ensure that the couple know how to work in any circumstances. If hospital-class contact and communication are not given adequate attention, I see a definite disadvantage to private classes.

I recently spoke to one of the student nurses who attend my classes. "I followed my case mother through labor last week," she told me. "She knew her breathing. But she and her husband didn't know how to work with hospital staff. When an intern came in and said she could have an epidural any time, she forgot all about the techniques and she had one, even though she didn't seem to need it. Tonight your husband was discussing with the men how to encourage the woman when that happens so that any medication will be her decision. But that woman's husband just didn't seem to know how to do that." This particular couple had attended a Lamaze class which I know to be quite a good one — except that there seems to be very little connection between the hospital situation and what the women are being taught.

On the pro side of classes conducted outside of the hospital, the atmosphere can be more informal and homey and the classes are usually considerably smaller — allowing ample opportunity for interaction between the couples. Community classes, given by public health clinics, colleges or community centres, can be excellent or mediocre — depending on how closely they work with the hospitals.

Classes Given by Non-Professionals:

These are usually given in conjunction with a professional or group of professionals. They can be extremely effective if given by a mother who has had a positive birth experience and who has completed some sort of preparation course, for example the course given by The American Society For Psychoprophylaxis In Obstetrics (ASPO). Graduates of this detailed, excellent teaching course are qualified to teach the Lamaze Method. Once again, the amount of communication with the medical community can determine their effectiveness.

Sometimes, a woman with no training gives classes — the only preparation being her use of the techniques for her own birth. These are possibly good classes,, but may tend to lack information on high risk pregnancies, complications and variations on normal labor.

Husband-Wife Teaching Teams:

In 1967 in Madison Wisconsin, under the direction of Dr. Sandra O'Leary, "Parentcraft" was formed. The difference between Parentcraft and other similar groups was that most teaching was done by couples in their own home. Instructors were required to:

1. have had one baby by the Lamaze method.
2. have breastfed one baby.
3. expect to be in Madison for two years.
4. be willing to teach as a couple.
5. be willing to teach at home.
6. have teaching and/or hospital experience.

In their pamphlet "Husband-Wife Teaching Teams In Childbirth Education", Karma and Michael Donnelly write, "Prospective teachers should write a resumé outlining their education and employment background and a statement of why they want to teach Lamaze classes and a labor and birth report. Usually the Parentcraft Committee looks at both husband and wife for an enthusiastic and genuinely positive attitude towards birth. When a couple is accepted for training they begin a course of training which lasts from four to six months."[1]

A class in which couples teach couples offers some obvious and immediate advantages. Right from the start, the expectant couple see the childbirth experience quite naturally as one for both man and woman. The man's teaching automatically puts the men at ease and helps clarify their role.

Unfortunately many of the husband-wife teaching teams have dropped out in Madison — partly because of additional time demands and pressures placed on the couple; and partly because for the man, childbirth education is rarely his occupation. Giving classes usually amounts to "moonlighting"; enthusiasm seems to wane as his children grow.

David and I have tried couple teaching and have found much the same problems. In classes held at home, usually there are small children around and the father supervises bedtime while his wife teaches. We've experienced the "the house is a shambles and the class is due in ten minutes and Tilke doesn't want to go to sleep and you're speaking tonight" chaos, which although giving the couples a view of normal family life, puts an undeniable strain on the couple who usually feel compelled to present a favorable view of parenthood.

I remember one awful evening when the baby refused to sleep, the movie projector broke and the dog escaped. Several of the fathers raced into the night to catch him, leaving me to nurse our new baby while David swore gently at the projector. Fifteen minutes later the fathers returned, triumphant. Unfortunately the dog they had cornered in the park and dragged home was not our Bogart. This particular class kept in touch with us for many months after the birth. They felt we needed support!

We've finally worked out an arrangement in which David takes one class in each series to discuss the man's role in pregnancy, birth and parenthood. It seems to be extremely successful. One man phoned and told me, "I have to fly out of town on business — if it's the men's class I'll cancel the appointment." It was and he did.

How to Choose a Childbirth Education Course

You've chosen your doctor carefully and are now looking for a course. Your doctor has possibly recommended the one given by the hospital. Most hospitals will send you a copy of the syllabus upon request. What do you look for?

Step One: Decide on the type of birth experience you want and choose a course which will prepare you for this.

For example, you, the father may decide that you would like to participate but not in every session. Look for a course which provides the woman for birth with basically psychoprophylactic techniques but where the father does not attend every session as "coach" — even though you may practice at home together. This sort of course is likely to be advertised as "Modified Lamaze", "Kitzinger Method" or "Read" method (the latter teaching a somewhat varying technique of psychoprophylaxis). "Erna Wright" or "Maternity Center Association" classes may or may not include the father at all sessions.

You, the woman may decide to take a course for women only. Most hospitals offer such courses, during the day, free. Evening courses tend to be more couple-oriented, but often require a fee.

If you have taken classes for the first baby (or second or third) and want a refresher course, a six-week series — commencing about eight weeks before birth, — should be adequate. If you are expecting your first child and want full preparation for pregnancy, birth and parenthood, your best bet is a course with early pregnancy and post partum sections, in addition to birth preparation.

Step two: Your doctor, whom you have chosen carefully, has referred you to a course, probably the classes at the hospital of his/her affiliation. Checking out this course will, incidentally, give you a fairly accurate idea of your doctor's views. Phone the hospital: usually the physiotherapy department of the obstetrical nursing office handles childbirth education. Ask if there is a printed prospectus of the course. Many hospitals have these and will usually send you one, or you can kill two birds with one stone and call in to pick up and arrange this to coincide with a hospital tour. (See Chapter 10.)

If you want couple-oriented childbirth or specifically Lamaze Method, choose your course carefully. Lamaze classes have become fashionable and many which are advertised as "Lamaze" are not really Lamaze, but general classes combining the principles of Read method with Lamaze.

If the hospital classes are advertised as Lamaze, try to arrange to sit in on one of the series in the birth preparation. This is not routine, but few hospitals would object. You'll learn a lot about the type of course by observing just one class. Are fathers actively involved in the class, or merely observing? Do they seem at ease? Are the couples enthusiastic (one of the results of truly couple-oriented classes)? Is there free discussion or does the instructor lecture formally and give little opportunity for the couples to participate? Does the instructor seem enthusiastic? (Extremely important!) Are many questions asked? When techniques are taught, is conditioning an integral part? Does the coach give consistent instructions to his partner, or is the practice haphazard? With Lamaze, usually you'll hear very definite, repeated instructions and the coach will do much of the teaching himself, after the new techniques have been shown.

Step Three: If you like the course, you're home and dry! But what if the course you're referred to isn't what you're looking for? Where do you go next? In many cities there is a branch of ICEA, which probably gives Lamaze classes. Make sure these classes are what you want by asking for printed material. Usually, instructors will be delighted to furnish you with this and invite you to observe a class. Perhaps you've heard of classes given by community services or private individuals. Phone and ask for information. Most private childbirth educators will furnish you with an outline of the course, the experience of the instructor and anything else you'd like to know. If the course is private, check to see what hospital communication there is: the instructor's background will give you a good idea of this. Most instructors will be able to give you some recommendations in writing from couples who have taken the course.

Step Four: Perhaps you've done quite a lot of shopping and finally come up with a course which sounds suitable. There are some other points to check.

- Is nutrition included? Who teaches it? Are films included?
- Is provision made for a hospital tour?
- Is provision made for revision classes until you have your child? If a course finishes five weeks before you give birth, you may lose incentive to practice your techniques. Even more critical, you miss the emotional support of the group — which most couples find invaluable at this time.
- Is there a post partum program?
- Is information on breastfeeding and the new baby included?
- If you specifically are aiming for a non-medicated birth, ask how many women usually do have no medication. This is certainly not a criterion for a good course, but it will give you some idea of how well the instructor supports PC. (In my own course, about 84% of women do not need medication.) Avoid the sort of course which teaches, "What to do until you have your epidural" — it's fine for some women but does not give encouragement to couples who do not want routine epidural.
- Smaller classes generally offer more personal attention and may be more conducive to open discussion and group interaction. If the class is large (more than ten couples), ask if the group divides into smaller groups. Generally, smaller classes have six to eight couples, medium-sized eight to twelve, and large classes more than twelve couples.

Cost

Ideally, every woman and her coach would have access to good, couple-oriented evening classes — free. Such classes are rare in North America, where even hospital-run courses may charge for evening classes.

In most Canadian cities, the free classes are usually held in the day only, thus eliminating not only most men, but working women also. Currently, with one exception only, evening courses in Montreal charge a fee, regardless of where they are given. The proposed plan in Quebec to provide government-run programs may solve this problem for many couples.

Does the course offer good value for your money? When comparing prices of various courses, consider the following factors: numbers of people in classes; whether it's oriented to women or couples; total number of hours of teaching; experience of instructor(s); number of people involved in teaching; use of audio-visual aids, printed notes, etc.

In most cities there are not enough couple-oriented programs — free or otherwise. It's the old cliché of supply and demand. Until doctors refer routinely to couple classes, the woman-centered class will continue to be the norm. As more and more couples ask for classes, more and more will be started.

In 1968 my course at the Catherine Booth Hospital was the only course for couples in the entire city. It was a Lamaze program, in the evening — and free. There were a few courses where fathers attended a "father's night", but none in which fathers attended each session. Since then I have helped start half a dozen new evening programs for couples and each year the number increases, many of them taught by graduates of my classes.

More demand produces more supply — more classes. To make choices about "methods", I'd recommend that you read as widely as possible, then start looking for a suitable course as soon as possible in pregnancy.

8 The right to a shared birth experience

Why would a father want to be there? Even the doctors are ashamed to be there — that's why they all wear masks, so's no-one will recognize them!
— *Archie Bunker,*
"All in the Family" TV series

Why indeed would a father want to join his mate in that mysterious and sterile inner sanctum, the "delivery room?" There may be blood, who knows what might go wrong, he's not a doctor and will probably feel out of place at this traditionally female event: he might be completely "turned off" by the gore and screaming, and even — horrors — might faint.

Yet every year many thousands of North American men participate in the birth of their children, and find this experience to be fascinating, fulfilling, and — something that may seem unbelievable — *sensual!* Typical of these is one of my clients, 25-year-old Ken Bresnen, prepared father of Jeremy, who believes that the father's presence at the birth of his child not only brings the couple closer, but may have far-reaching effects on family life:

> *I was not turned off by anything in the birth and I don't regard myself as particularly strong stomached. But I wouldn't have missed it for anything. During the labor, I was too busy coaching my wife to even think of fainting. Since then, our love has grown to the point where I wonder how I can express it all! We conceived our child together, it was natural that we'd experience birth together. I felt close to my son right from birth. I naturally take an active part in his care and I believe that this will have a significant bearing on our relationship when he's older.*

Childbirth as Ecstasy?

Author of *Husband-Coached Childbirth,* Dr. Robert Bradley agrees that birth is an expression of love at its finest. He writes:

> *I include the father because there is simply no substitute for him. . . I had observed for years that women seemed to fall in love with their obstetricians. This says nothing about the loveableness of the obstetrician: it's because bearing a child is a love act in itself. . . people watching husband-coached childbirth often say that they feel like intruders in a room where a man and a woman are making love. It's joyful to the point of ecstasy.* [1]

I would certainly agree with his observation. Physiologically, the changes as a woman approaches birth are almost identical to the process leading to orgasm. I have frequently heard women approaching the moment of birth vocalize as in the act of love. I remember prominent anthropologist and childbirth educator, Sheila Kitzinger, addressing the conference of the International Childbirth

Education Association in 1972. "I believe in the pleasure principle in childbirth. When I was giving birth to my fifth child I remember saying over and over, 'Oh, it's such a lovely feeling . . . oh, it's such a lovely feeling!' "

Although this feeling of ecstasy happens frequently where the couple share birth, I have rarely seen a woman express the same emotion when the father was not present. His reassurance is the factor most important in helping her relax and fully experience birth. And unfortunately, the sexual quality of childbirth is all too often blunted — or eliminated — by hospital routines.

In the summer of 1975, David and I were invited to conduct a three-hour workshop at Concordia University, Montreal, on "Childbirth and Sexuality". Although childbirth is so obviously a sexual experience in that it is centered around the sexual organs, few people in our culture would describe it as such. This attitude is partly caused by the fear and tension which too often surround birth, and partly by the constant interference with normal birth by innumerable procedures and routines. We wanted to illustrate how this interference might take the sensual punch out of a hospital birth so we invented the following game.

We had the group stand on one leg and raise the left arm high above the head and imagine that they were women experiencing labor. While I moderated the course of a normal labor, David walked from one to another and interfered constantly: "We're just going to give you an enema. Please ask your husband to step outside. Keep your arm still, we're just going to set up your IV. We're going to hook you up to the fetal monitor, try not to move so much . . . What was the date of your last menstrual period? Your mother's maiden name? Now we're just going to examine you. This is a little something to take the edge off things . . . Don't push yet, your doctor's not here. We're just washing you down . . . Push into your bottom as though you're having a big bowel movement. We're giving your baby a little help with forceps. You have a lovely baby. Don't touch!' "

Sensual? The point was well made, we felt. In these circumstances it is difficult for even the well prepared couple to think of birth as sensual — yet surprisingly, even under such clinical conditions many couples do manage to enjoy birth. That childbirth can for many women still be a sensual experience despite hospital management is indicative of the tremendous emotional bond between the man and woman throughout birth. Couples who work together during labor and share the birth frequently describe their experience as "the most beautiful sort of love relationship" and "an incredible peak of ecstasy." After all, birth is the final act in the sexual drama, the completion of the natural cycle from courting to conception to childbirth.

Robert H. Stewart, a Seattle physician, is one doctor who violently opposes the theory of birth as sensual. He writes:

> The male attitude to the female genitalia is one of unconscious hostility. To him the charm of a woman is her mystery. It is inconceivable that a normal male watching the delivery of his wife would experience anything but revulsion at the vision of these genitalia under the worst and filthiest conditions. [2]

"That man has entirely a warped notion of love," Tim Bradley replied angrily when a group of fathers discussed the quote. "All the way through Bev's birth I kept thinking how much I loved her, and I really feel it was one of the high points of our love. When you've shared the pregnancy as intimately as we did, then worked so hard together to give birth to your child, I think it comes naturally."

"I agree," said Ken Bresnen. "There has to be that emotional growth. I think if I hadn't had much to do with Ruth's pregnancy and had just walked into the birth, it wouldn't have been such a powerful experience. But it doesn't come easily. You have to work together to get it."

One quality of home birth which has impressed me greatly is its sensuality. Without interference, in familiar surroundings, the father close and uninhibited, birth can be more easily a sensual experience. I spoke to a young radio announcer some time ago, while we were preparing a program on couples' rights. He and his wife had had their baby at home because he was afraid he wouldn't be able to share fully in a hospital birth. "By home birth I don't mean that we didn't prepare fully — we were fully prepared and had medical attendance, but it was so calm and unhurried. My wife had orgasm at the moment of birth and it was unbelievably close and moving for both of us." Other couples I have discussed this with have agreed that home birth can be extremely sensual, yet this is possible also in a supportive hospital context.

Why Some Doctors Say No

When we began the Montreal Childbirth Education Association movement to open delivery rooms to fathers, we encountered plenty of objections. Obstetricians' opposition ranged from medical grounds to purely emotional arguments. It took several years of constant pressure from hundreds of men and women before Montreal's largest teaching hospital gave in and allowed fathers to attend the births of their children.

Before the policy about-face, I was present at this hospital to coach a friend's labor. At that time, the restrictions against fathers were so severe that her husband, Michael, a pediatric resident at the hospital, was not permitted in the delivery room. As labor progressed, Michael became increasingly involved and very much wanted to attend the delivery. He decided to go and seek dispensation from the obstetrical chief. He was familiar with the chief's views on fathers but felt he had nothing to lose. About fifteen minutes later, Michael returned, puffing furiously up the stairs — having been told that birth was a matter between a woman and her doctor and what sort of "dirty, disgusting man" would want to be present at his wife's birth? Michael decided he was just such a man and attended anyway, holding his wife's head as she delivered their daughter, laughing and crying with joy. I've never forgotten that birth: I was leaving for my wedding in Vermont in an hour and that little girl's glorious arrival seemed to be a good omen.

In the Montreal hospitals, other objections to a shared delivery included: "The father will get in the way" . . . "If I have to worry about the father I can't concentrate on the delivery" and "What sort of a man would want to?"

Medical arguments were more clearly defined and easier to disprove. The case against fathers was summed up as "increased risk or infection, increased risk of malpractice suit, and risk of the father's misconduct (collapsing or attacking the doctor!)."

What about these objections? Dr. Murray Enkin, Associate Professor at McMaster University and former Chief of Obstetrics and Gynecology at St. Joseph's Hospital in Hamilton, Ontario, introduced psychoprophylactic preparation for couples to St. Joseph's in 1964. Fathers are included routinely as active participants in the birth. Dr. Enkin says, "We have found no difficulties with the father's presence in the delivery room at any time." He counters another often-heard objection. "We have found no reason to exclude him from cases where epidurals are used or operative deliveries are carried out. In those instances where something goes wrong — a congenital abnormalcy, for example — his presence is invaluable. We have carefully monitored infection rates and bacterial colonization rates in the newborn and there has been no increase."[3]

One California survey published in 1971 shows that in more than 4,425 cases where the prepared father attended delivery there was not one single infection traceable to the practice, not a single malpractice suit, nor one case of a father's "misconduct".[4]

I have been present at hundreds of shared births but not once have I seen a prepared father faint, collapse or do anything other than embrace his partner and share the joy. Possibly the totally unprepared father standing there as a spectator might feel faint. But as Ken Bresnen noted, the prepared father is too busy for any of that!

As the formal objections have been dispelled and the father's presence at birth has become accepted at many hospitals, more and more doctors are discovering the benefits to the woman, the man and the staff: less anxiety; increased co-operation on the part of the woman; and more satisfaction for a doctor concerned with the well-being of the family.

One of the first obstetricians to recognize the benefits of father participation was Dr. Pierre Vellay of Paris. In a brief on "Husbands In The Delivery Room" published by the International Childbirth Education Association in 1965, he writes:

> *During pregnancy and preparation for confinement, the husband is an effective manager. He is, moreover, a link between his wife and the obstetrical team. This intimate collaboration . . . reinforces the bonds between the couple and their future child. The attention of the husband, his understanding, his kindness, enormously facilitates the pregnancy of his wife . . . The presence of the husband develops in him a feeling of paternity towards his child, which he will strive to assume to the utmost later on.[5]*

This feeling of paternity was the pervading spirit at an MCEA meeting in 1974 which we called "Men and Maternity". About three hundred couples (and assorted singles) listened as David discussed the man's role in pregnancy, childbirth and parenting with a panel of four fathers. Not one of the men had initially wanted to attend the birth of his child; none had foreseen that he would be involved in parenting to the extent which he obviously is. All of the men attended the birth because they wanted to, and all felt that they had been able to help their partners. Without exception they were extremely positive about their presence at the birth. "I really think the staff appreciated my help, because they thanked me afterwards," one said. All of the men agreed enthusiastically that active participation in pregnancy and birth had led to an unexpected intimate involvement with their children. These men are sharing parenting with considerable pleasure. Yet too often our social mores suppress a father's close involvement with his baby.

Human Fatherhood — A Social Invention?

At its best, father-coached childbirth does not end with the birth of the child — far from it. More and more I see fathers taking on what have traditionally been regarded as women's tasks in child-rearing. Though perhaps there is not yet a househusband on every suburban block, scarcely a single home with young children in residence exists where the father doesn't routinely perform jobs which his father would almost certainly have viewed as "woman's work". Today, fathers change diapers, fix formula and do bottle feedings, back pat, sing, soothe and coo with the best of mothers. Many are not beyond bathing the infant or even washing out the children's underthings.

That fathers are taking a new and active interest in parenting is beyond question. What is less clear is whether or not child care comes as naturally to men as it supposedly does to woman or whether — as with olives and anchovies — it is an acquired taste. In my opinion, men "mother" just as well as women. Furthermore, I believe that they have a natural bent in this direction: if society accepts a more intimate male-child role as normal, these usually locked-up instincts will come to the fore.

To test this idea, I went to the social and historical literature on childbirth. Thousands of words have been written on the subject from the starkly scientific to the mythic, but by and large they concentrate on the female. Too often, I was appalled to discover, writers either dispatch the man on a hunting or drinking party, give him some obscure tribal or religious function or forget him altogether while the women of the community get on with the blessed event.

There are of course some happy exceptions including this ray of hope from eminent anthropologist Margaret Mead, who writes in her book *Male And Female:*

> *It is perhaps not without significance that in those Polynesian societies where the male participates in his wife's delivery as a husband, not as a magician or priest, there is an extremely simple, uncomplicated attitude toward birth; women do not scream, but instead work, and men need no self-imposed expiatory activities afterward.*[6]

More encouraging still, Mead is at pains to remark on the extreme stability of these particular societies. But this helpful Polynesian chap is in marked contrast to the man of the Manus tribe Mead observed in New Guinea whom society forbids from taking an active role in childbirth. In *Growing Up In New Guinea,* Mead describes his predicament: "From the moment her labor begins . . . the father . . . may not see her. The nearest approach he can make to her house is to bring fish to the landing platform. For a whole month he wanders aimlessly about..." With such shabby treatment of the father it comes as little surprise to read that in this society, "the relationship between husband and wife is strained and cold."[7]

Much of what has been written on father participation describes the *couvade* — a custom found in many parts of the world in which the father acts as though he were in labor. In some cases, he may even be put to bed and cared for until after the birth.

There is more to this custom than its being merely a quaint custom on the part of primitives. A recent report published in the *British Journal of Psychiatry* entitled "The Couvade Syndrome" discovered that men often do experience symptoms similar to those of their pregnant mates. The study concluded "that possibly one in nine males may have some symptoms of psychogenic origin in relation to their partners' pregnancies."[8] Another survey, conducted in Washington, D. C. and still being evaluated, suggests that as many as 65% of men with pregnant mates experience bloating, nausea, abdominal cramps and sensations similar to labor "pains".[9] These studies suggest that there is a direct physical link between men and maternity. Possibly the current interest of men in birth and parenting merely revives instincts lost in our ancient past!

I believe very strongly that the North American movement toward active father participation in childbirth and early family life will enormously benefit Western society. Since the 1920's, an increasing number of sociologists have decried the decline of the family in this culture, suggesting that it portends the fall of the West. (Prior to the 20's, interestingly, many men did participate in birth — a fairly simple procedure at a time when home birth was common). Certainly, the huge pressures of the post-industrial world in which we live and work have, until recently, been divisive. Currently, many men seem to be retreating into the comfort of a smoothly functioning family. This retreat may well be a reaction to the mechanization of the age: I believe it may also prove to be a key factor in the ultimate greening of North America.

My experiences with thousands of couples who have shared intimately their thoughts and emotions from conception, through pregnancy to the birth of their child are disproving the traditional idea that fathering is simply "providing". (Mead believes that "human fatherhood is a social invention" and that "men have to want to learn to provide for others and this behaviour being learned is fragile and can disappear rather easily under social conditions that no longer teach it effectively.")[10] Rather than merely providing, each week at my parenting classes fathers experience genuine pleasure in baby care, in tenderness and in close physical contact with their young. As a result of these sessions, I now believe that fathers who share pregnancy and birth with their partners are more likely to derive real pleasure from child care than those who are isolated from the childbearing experience.

Traditional roles are being challenged today. Many of my

couples share child care and careers, although this feat is still difficult in our society. The more equal joint parenting I see in these couples is, I believe, the result of a close bonding at the time of birth. Women who are deprived of close contact with their babies at birth may show weakened mothering behaviour (see Chaper 10) and on the same basis, men who are excluded from birth may show weak fathering patterns. Conversely, when both parents share the birth, a strong parenting instinct is nurtured in both man and woman. To allow men to participate and enjoy what have traditionally been regarded as female areas is part of human liberation — as necessary to the liberation of men as equal salaries and career opportunities are to the liberation of women.

The role of the pregnant father in our culture has for too long been portrayed as that of doddering midnight pickle hunter, butt of countless jokes: the lovable buffoon roaring in panic to the hospital with his laboring partner at ninety miles an hour; the chain smoking wretch pacing the waiting room; the self-conscious bumbler fumbling out the cigars. Later, he becomes the man who busies himself with a career because there is no place for him in the care of his baby; the man who drifts away from his wife because they no longer have much in common. There is little in these traditions to create the image of a man strong and competent. It is easy to see how "momism" has developed — a disservice both to man and woman. These false and misleading stereotypes imply that fathers are not to be trusted with baby care!

Some current writers believe that most men are not interested in fathering. Pamela Mason writes in *Marriage Is The First Step to Divorce:*

> *The male animal . . . really has very little interest in watching his young grow up, unless he's having a marvellous time with the female who provided him with the young. Often, by the time the young have grown up, he has another female who is also giving him a marvellous time and more young to grow up. Sometimes he's very*

*clever and gets a female who doesn't have any young at
all. Then he's much happier altogether. [11]*

According to this reasoning, it's remarkable that the race
has lasted this long. What rubbish! Every man of course has
moments when he is slightly less fond of children than was W.
C. Fields ("Show me a man who hates kids and I'll show you
a man who can't be all bad.") But what woman is eternally
devoted to her children, never short tempered, always loving?
Whether we like it or not, there is a difference between the
worlds of adult and child. Ms. Mason uses these natural differences to denigrate both sexes.

My experience has been quite different. Many of the men in
my classs are fathering second families — of these, most
openly admit that they're enjoying the second parenting
more, because of their close involvement with the whole
process. They're having a "marvelous time" with the baby,
not in spite of it. Peter recently shared the birth of his
daughter. During his first marriage he fathered two children
without becoming involved in the process. He now believes
that sharing pregnancy, birth and parenting is the only way to
be a father:

> *With my first marriage, I didn't know a thing about
> childbirth . . . I was busy trying to get ahead in my job.
> I spent the whole birth doing that horrible pacing out-
> side and feeling guilty for putting my wife through it all.
> After our son was born she told me "Never again."
> Neither of us knew a thing about babies. My wife was
> stuck at home while I spent long hours at the office.*
>
> *I'd come home from work and find my wife in tears,
> but I just didn't want to hear about her problems. When
> I did do anything with the baby she'd tell me I was doing
> it all wrong, so I started leaving all the baby care to her.*
>
> *When the second baby was born, it was a repeat of
> the first time except that my wife was more competent
> . . . Finally after four years we decided that we didn't*

*have a thing in common — my wife resented being just a
mother but felt she had no other role in life . . . We
divorced.*

*With this baby it was so different . . . I didn't want to
have anything to do with the birth at first but then I
decided that if I were going to have another child I wanted to share. I look forward to getting home to play with
the baby each day. Even when it's rough — you're both
exhausted and irritable, the baby has been awake all
night — it's more fun because we can talk about it and
we can share the baby. I'm sure that if we'd done things
this way, my first marriage would have been better. You
get out of parenting what you put in, but most men
don't know and aren't given the chance to put in.*

Men and Childbirth Classes

Most pregnant fathers arrive at my initial class somewhat
ill at ease and clearly wishing they were elsewhere. The more
positive ones are usually those who have been recommended
to the course by friends. Often those men who have had
children before but did not participate are the most eager to
share this time. Any uneasiness vanishes as it quickly becomes
apparent to the men that the father's role in pregnancy, birth
and parenting is a vitally important one.

A course which is couple-oriented does not simply "include" the father, but gears much of the teaching to his
needs. In a good childbirth education class, man and woman
are viewed as a closely-knit team.

One of the more gratifying aspects of couple classes is the
communication which gradually develops between not only
each couple but among the couples in the group. It's
reassuring to discuss feelings and changes with other men and
women. By the time of the actual birth experience (or as a
physiotherapy student taking my course replied on an exam
paper, the "experiment"), men are usually completely
engrossed and enthusiastic about participation.

The shared birth experience, I believe, should include the

father in every phase of the labor, birth and post partum period, should he and his partner wish. Many couples would prefer to remain together during admissions, preps, internals as well as birth. In other countries the role of the "monitrice" or labor "coach" is accepted as essential to the woman's physical and emotional comfort. There is no question of the monitrice not staying for everything. In North America, it's ironic that the father-as-coach concept began out of need, a result of the lack of monitrices — but it's turned into a radical innovation which has changed the centuries-old notion that childbirth is for women, and their attendant midwives or doctors. As well, the entry of the father into the delivery room has changed and enriched the relationship of women and their mates, and possibly the relationships of men and their children.

If fathers are to be "coaches" in the full sense of the word, they must be allowed to coach at all times. Bill Mann in Chapter 3 remained with Jean during admission, internals, labor and delivery. So did David S.:

> *I simply asked our doctor if I could and he told me that he didn't have any objections. When I got to the hospital I used his promise a lot. Several people came in and asked me to leave, but each time I explained that I had permission to stay and I realized that it wasn't routine but would they mind? Nobody minded and after a while the staff made sure that when someone new came in they told him, "that father stays."*

Coping With the Reluctant Father

"Honey, I've played midwife to enough cows in my life to know what it's all about. I've had my arm in cows up to the elbows trying to deliver a calf. If it's just the same with you, I'd rather not be present," one man I know told his wife. How do you deal with a mate who blanches at the suggestion of attending a single prenatal class — much less coaching you in the delivery room? In my experience, even the most reluctant father becomes enthusiastic when he realizes that he is an essential part of the birth process. The trick seems to be to get him to the first class — and to make sure that this class is geared to the father as well as the mother. It helps if you choose a course in which all of the fathers routinely attend, and the atmosphere is relaxed and informal.

I would suggest you use the following approach. "All I ask is that you come with me to one class. If you really feel afterwards that it's not for you, okay — I'll understand. But I'm determined to use PC, and if you don't feel up to it, I'll use a friend." If one class doesn't generate some interest in him, by all means ask a close friend to act as coach. A friend can also be a good stand-by coach if your mate travels frequently and there's a possibility he may be out of town when your baby is born.

For almost every prepared father — even the previously reluctant one — the birth experience is a growing, positive one. Sometimes such a growth is dramatic. Sherry came to classes with a woman friend to coach her. Luke, the baby's father showed no interest — in fact, he was extremely negative. On the fourth evening he arrived alone, and sat in a corner looking uneasy and not saying a word. The following week Sherry came with Luke. He began to coach. The following week, he asked many questions. In the weeks that followed, Luke became an interested and active member of the group. After the birth he phoned me excitedly, "We did it!" It had been wonderful, he said: he and Sherry had worked together throughout.

Several months after the birth Luke assumed daily care of the baby while Sherry returned to her job. They both seemed comfortable with this arrangement. I came into the living room one night to overhear my husband, David speaking to someone on the phone, in a conversation peppered with the in-talk of a confirmed child raiser. "Oh, that was Luke, the baby has diarrhea!" The two fathers engaged in several of these conversations, earnestly and with fatherly concern, and Luke is not an isolated example.

Penny came to classes without her husband who simply refused to have anything to do with any part of it. I coached her until almost the end of the course. Then John came one night to collect her. He sat in on the end of the class and the following week came with her. I had assured Penny that I would coach her through labor, but my offer turned out to be unnecessary. I did attend the birth, but as a friend rather than a coach. John took over completely, took photos and was the first to cuddle their son.

Recently Penny and John came in for their second child. Once more I attended as a friend. John coached again and was obviously proud. He and Penny share the raising of the two boys and I believe that their shared births certainly helped.

Complications and Caesarean Births

What of complicated and Caesarean births? In both cases the father's role can be tremendously helpful in the support and encouragement of the woman. I have watched fathers present at difficult deliveries helping their wives by constantly encouraging — working with the medical staff. In every one of these complicated deliveries, the father's loving and reassuring presence served only to help the mother.

Many hospitals have accepted the father's presence for normal births, but may draw the line at his observing Caesarean birth. However, many "C-sections" today are performed under epidural anesthetic; and the woman, although screened off from the actual operation, can hear the baby cry and be shown it from the start. Some doctors, such as Murray Enkin, have included the father at some Caesarean births with only positive results. "I never exclude the father if he wants to be present," Dr. Enkin told me.

Paul Walker attended the Caesarean birth of his son, pre-arranged with the doctor, who knew in advance that Caesarean would be necessary. In the Baltimore Childbirth Education Association newsletter, 1973, he writes:

*I realized afterwards how disappointed I would have
been to have totally missed our baby's birth . . . My
being there gave me a perspective my wife could never
have described and by telling her what she herself could
not see I helped make the experience more total for her
. . . Sharing our son's cry with my wife was an inde-
scribable experience.*

Among my clients, the few fathers who have attended
Caesarean agree with him, and their wives speak of the
tremendous support in having them present.

Do-It-Yourself Delivery

One recent development in the father participation field has
been initiated by Dr. William Hazlett in Kingston, Penn-
sylvania, who teaches the father to deliver the baby himself.
Hazlett at first questioned the use of the epidural because,
"The mother had no sensation and was unable to play any
role in the actual birth." He adds, "Women weren't getting
much kick out of childbirth." In 1955 he gave up spinals,
using a sedative where necessary and a local when he deems
episiotomy necessary.

In 1968, Hazlett agreed to let a father deliver his third
child: it worked so well that he now routinely supervises the
father. When the father requests it, about a month before
delivery, Dr. Hazlett instructs him in normal delivery
technique. When the time comes, Hazlett supervises the birth
but does not intervene unless there are complications. Of particular concern to Hazlett is the depersonalization and
mechanization of obstetrics. He says that he is concerned that
all the equipment now used in delivery rooms may eventually
force the father out. "I think that would be a mistake — each
man needs to have his own special experience at the birth of a
child."[12]

Managing editor of the Canadian magazine, *Saturday
Night,* Robert Fulford managed to have his own special experience, but only after two previous births in which this was

denied him. Although Fulford's "special experience" did not include delivering his child, it was so fulfilling that in an article in *Chatelaine* Magazine, December 1972, entitled, "Letter To A Pregnant Father" he writes:

> *Be there when it happens. Right now, get on the phone to your wife's obstetrician and find out if you can be in the delivery room. Don't accept a maybe — get him or her to promise you'll be there. If he won't promise, make your wife change doctors. If you don't, you'll be cheating yourself of one of the great moments of your life . . . During the two deliveries of my previous marriage I did that awful business of pacing up and down the corridors imagining God knows what, accepting it as the way it had to be. Since the new baby I've developed a deep resentment of all doctors and hospitals who high-handedly ban fathers from the delivery room and deny them this experience.*

I believe that denying the father participation is denying the couple their right to a necessary growth experience. It is often said that the strength of a society is equal to the strength of the family. Shared childbirth, I feel, is a vitally important factor in the strength of the family.

The Right To A "Coach"

Every woman has the right to constant emotional support throughout labor. I have watched births in several other countries where a nurse or midwife sat with the woman for the entire labor, encouraging her and making her comfortable. And I have watched too many births in this country where the unfortunate woman, — without a husband or friend to coach — suffered alone in a small cubicle for the seemingly endless hours of labor. The nurse checked her routinely, but because she was busy with other things could not stay with her all the time.

The single mother is often badly neglected on our maternity

wards; she frequently becomes a teaching subject for students, and obstetrical procedures of dubious necessity may be used on her, often without explanation. I have coached many single women through labor: some were prepared, but most were very young, totally unprepared and frightened. (One fifteen-year-old that I accompanied through labor confessed that she was terrified of dying in childbirth). The mere presence of someone throughout labor can prevent physical and emotional suffering, regardless of whether the woman is prepared or not.

In the summer of 1975 I organized, through a women's group, the first program in Montreal to prepare single women for birth in the psychoprophylactic method. Assisted by volunteers, I found and trained women as coaches who would practice with their partners and accompany them throughout the birth. Although there was difficulty matching the coaches to the women, it was a successful program, which has since been followed by other centers in the city.

But many hospitals refuse to believe in the woman's right to a coach — particularly if she is single. One woman coach told me:

> The labor went smoothly and my partner was in full control, but when it came time for delivery I was told I'd have to stay outside "Because you're not the baby's father!" I tried to speak to the head nurse but it was too late and my partner lost her control. That wouldn't have happened if I'd been allowed in. I felt they were discriminating against her.

As in other countries, a nurse could be specifically assigned to the single woman; or courses can prepare a coach, a friend or volunteer coach, to accompany her through labor.

Thoughts On Shared Childbirth

> Gareth was an incredible strength and support. It was

an experience we shall both treasure. "

— Carol

The most important part was feeling that Natalie was born months before delivery. The sharing and closeness is quite extraordinary. The preparation gave us the opportunity to appreciate the total experience with far more depth than I'd expected.

— Gareth

Throughout labor I knew that we were prepared for and aware of all that was happening.

— Heather

I was amazed at how efficient the training was. The rapport that exists between my wife and me towards the baby is amazing.

— Gilles

How To Make Sure You're Together

I firmly believe that parents should be able to share each phase of labor and birth, not as a privilege but as a right. Words such as "allow" and "permit" miss the heart of the matter. The word "include" would be the obvious choice — but we have a long way to go before the father is automatically included instead of being "permitted" or tolerated.

To date, there is no legally defined right to shared childbirth. But in 1973 a bill was presented to the United States Congress by Martha Griffiths (D-Mich.) guaranteeing the father's right to attend the birth of his child if the mother agrees. It read:

Be it enacted by the Senate and House of Representatives of the United States of America . . . that any hospital, clinic or similar establishment set up for the purpose of fostering, restoring or observing a person's

*health and which receives Federal funds . . . shall allow
the biological father to be in attendance during all
phases of childbirth if consent is first obtained from the
woman involved. [13]*

The bill was never passed. And although in the U.S., a
number of parents have taken hospitals to court in an attempt
to permit father-coached childbirth, these lawsuits have been
universally unsuccessful as we go to press. Writing in the
Medicolegal News, George J. Annas, J.D., M.P.H., of the
Boston University School of Medicine, says of one appellate
decision:

*While conceding that "the birth of a child is an event of
unequalled importance in the lives of most married
couples," the court found the birth procedure itself . . .
to be "comparable to other serious hospital procedures," and "extraordinary" in nature. This, of
course, rejects the entire rationale of the (prepared)
childbirth movement, which is that childbirth is natural,
not pathological, and that in the vast majority of births
little or no medical intervention is either required or
desirable . . .*

*While minor victories in this battle may be won in the
courts, civil litigation, as illustrated by the "father in
the delivery room cases" is not a terribly effective way
of promoting safe alternatives to present childbirth
methods. The proper arenas are likely to be the . . .
legislatures and health regulatory agencies, and the
proper issue is patient influence on the way childbirth
services are delivered. [14]*

I hope that father participation may be a legally defined
right throughout North America at some time in the future.
Meanwhile, you can virtually guarantee yourself a shared
childbirth — providing there are no complications — if you
use the following system.

1. Choose your doctor carefully. (See Chapter 5.) Both of
    you should go to a prenatal check up — the first if
    possible — and discuss being together with the doctor.
    Ask about colleagues. If your doctor assures you that all
    the doctors in his/her group allow or include the father
    routinely, then you've probably not a concern in the
    world. If however, your doctor hedges about some of the
    group you may be in trouble. Pin him/her down to a
    definite answer. If you're told that Dr. B. sometimes will
    not include the father, at least you know where you
    stand. You can either take the chance that you may or
    may not have Dr. B., or you can explain to your doctor
    that in such an important matter you'd rather not take
    any chances — and look for another group. Remember,
    you probably only experience childbirth once or twice in
    your life: nothing is worth making a compromise over
    being together if that's what you want!
2. The doctor says that he usually "permits" the father to
    attend. Try to find out under what conditions he/she
    doesn't. If it's "if we're busy, if there's a complication
    . . ." from my experience that probably means "there's a
    very good chance that at the slightest excuse I'll say no."
    If you can't get a satisfactory answer, you'll probably
    feel better with a doctor who does not just tolerate
    fathers but who is enthusiastic about having them at birth.
    There are plenty of these around: once doctors in-
    clude the father, they usually become converts. "It's
    more fun," says one doctor. "You're dealing with
    people, not patients when you have both members of the
    couple there. I think it makes me pay more attention to
    the woman as a person too, when her husband is there."
3. Discuss the father's being there in case of complication or
    in the case of Caesarean birth, if regional (epidural)
    anesthetic is used. Also ask about your doctor's preferen-
    ces in anesthesia in case of complications. By bringing up
    the subject, you may help to make shared Caesarean with
    epidural (rather than general anesthetic) routine.

4. Discuss the possibility of the father's being present during admissions, prepping and internal examinations, if you wish. Your doctor probably won't be there at the time, but having his/her permission goes a long way.

5. During childbirth, if for some reason, the father is excluded, both of you should ask for a definite reason. If there doesn't seem to be one, demand an explanation. Use all the ammunition you have — including the fact that the doctor promised you could be together. This is one time when you can *demand*. If you don't, you may miss an experience which you may never be able to repeat.

   Note to father: In extreme cases, if all else fails and your doctor has given permission, JUST GET IN THE DELIVERY ROOM!

With any luck, your situation won't be this drastic, but here's how two couples made sure they were together:

Joan and Ed had their doctor's permission to be together during the birth. A colleague was on duty. He turned to Ed just as the nurses were getting ready to take Joan to the delivery room and said, "I'm sorry but I'd rather you didn't come. Fathers make me nervous." Joan thought quickly. "Then I hope you're ready to deliver in this bed, because I'm not going anywhere if Ed isn't with me. Could you get the resident?" The nurses rallied and found the resident; Joan, Ed, the nurses and the resident filed into the delivery room, and fifteen minutes later the baby arrived. Not exactly an ideal situation — but they were together as they had been promised they would be.

Panny and Bob arrived at the hospital when Panny was close to birth. It was her second child and this one was coming quickly. She was taken straight into the delivery room. Bob was told that labor was going too quickly and he'd have to wait because the doctor wasn't there. Bob had been to the hospital tour the previous week and knew where to change. He whisked into delivery room garb and was as Panny's side in five minutes helping her push. Nobody threw him out. The doctor never did make it, but with Bob's coaching Panny remained calm as a nurse attended the birth. Chapter 11 outlines more UPC techniques of dealing with staff to ensure you get shared childbirth. But most hospital hassles can be avoided if you choose your doctor carefully, and communicate effectively with him or her beforehand. REMEMBER — IT'S BETTER TO DISCUSS EVERYTHING WITH YOUR DOCTOR LONG IN ADVANCE THAN DURING LABOR!

9 The right to childbirth with dignity

When I arrived at the hospital my labor was very strong and on examination they found my cervix was 6 centimeters dilated. I'd had a large bowel movement at home and asked to skip the enema because I was afraid it would throw my concentration. The nurse told me that it was "policy" to give every woman an enema and insisted on giving me one. They wouldn't let Bill stay with me, because of "policy" and they treated us like a pair of tiresome school kids. After the enema they insisted on setting up an IV and the fetal monitor, and didn't even answer when I asked whether that was absolutely necessary.

By this time I had the urge to push and asked to be examined. They told me I couldn't possibly be ready to deliver, but the urge was so strong that finally I yelled. The resident confirmed what I knew — that my cervix was fully dilated. My own doctor wasn't around and they told me he'd ordered an epidural. I didn't want one but they said he thought it would be needed for delivery.

> *The epidural seemed to slow everything down, and I'm sure that it was to give the doctor time to get there.*
>
> *When he arrived, he performed what I felt was a routine forceps delivery. I was left feeling that I was the last person to have any say in how my daughter was born.*
>
> *—Emily*

My files bulge with letters resembling Emily's — from couples angry with their treatment during childbirth. "I felt like an animal" . . . "They treated me like a piece of meat" . . . "It was as if I didn't have a brain, or any feelings at all. Surely it must be possible to have childbirth with dignity!"

It may at first seem laughable — to speak of dignity when a woman is in the unladylike position of childbirth. But I believe that the woman who is in control of her body can accomplish childbirth with a sense of true self-respect and esteem.

I believe that all pregnant parents have the right to choose a hospital which will allow them flexibility in the way in which they have their babies. In delivery, the woman must be allowed to choose the position in which she feels most comfortable — and she must be supported by the staff in her choice. The hospital should not insist on routine procedures — such as prepping, separating the couple during admission, lithotomy position, anesthetic, induction, strapping of hands and use of stirrups, episiotomy, and separating mother and infant after birth — simply because of hospital policy. Childbirth with dignity means allowing the couple reasonable choice in the way their child is born. It's respecting their wishes and allowing them some degree of decision making. It centers on the needs of the clients, rather than on staff, and avoids unnecessary routines performed in the name of hospital "policy". It's as one wonderful head nurse once said to me, the right to give birth as you choose: "If the couple want to chant and sing and burn incense and have the baby squatting, that's fine with me!" A rare and compassionate nurse who was as good as her word.

Perhaps if the word "client" were to replace the word "patient", childbirth with dignity would be routine. The word "patient" conjures up a roomful of women, in late pregnancy, waiting "patiently" for up to an hour, sometimes longer for a three minute, "You're fine" and being grateful for that! Let's imagine for a moment that you're visiting a hairdresser: Few salons would stay in business if clients were expected routinely to sit around for an hour or so for an appointment they were told was an hour ago. Let's take the analogy a little further. You ask the hairdresser to give you curls. He replies "Sorry, but waves are salon policy!" An outlandish answer to a reasonable request. But no more outlandish than what happens in hospital when a woman reasonably asks for a clip in place of a shave, or no enema when she's already had a bowel movement, or a simple variation in birth position. Thus, childbirth with dignity is a client-oriented birth experience.

Many hospital routines exist only because of hospital "policy" — an attempt to make all couples conform to certain procedures. Such routines, discussed in Chapter 3, have been proven conclusively to be not in the best interests of either mother or baby. A client-oriented hospital grants flexible choices in the way in which labor and birth proceed, and assesses the need for procedures on an individual basis rather than that of policy.

But it's more than just routines and procedures. In a truly client-oriented childbirth, the staff actively supports and respects the couple's choices — as long as these choices are reasonable. Staff attitudes can contribute immensely to whether the experience is dignified or otherwise. For example, three couples recently arrived at my class, distressed about the hospital tour they had been given the previous evening.

"We'd heard good things about our hospital, but it's hard to believe them now," Judy K. told me. "The nurse who was giving the tour took us into the labor room and said, 'Here's where you'll spend your hours of agony!' Maybe it was her idea of a joke, but she sure wasn't funny . . ."

Her husband Allen continued, "She told us that the father would absolutely not be allowed to enter the delivery room until the doctor arrived. Anyhow, she said, the father's main job was to get the nurse when she was needed. She told me, 'You don't really have much to do — you'll be changing the pads under your wife, but that's about all.' "

"In the delivery room, she said, 'There's nothing ladylike about this room! No way around it, childbirth really hurts!' " Sharon O. complained. "We asked about stirrups and she told us they were mandatory. And when I asked about having the baby right after birth, she said I'd have to wait eight hours or more . . ."

Allen K. added that the anesthetist had compounded the nurse's damage. "He showed me a lot of photos of women with epidurals . . . as though a woman couldn't have a baby without one and we should all be thankful to him."

Horrified, I pointed out that this nurse's views did not reflect the general approach of the hospital at all. The previous week, several couples who had given birth there had praised the flexible, supportive, caring staff — all of these couples had been given their babies right after birth. I suggested that the three couples write to the supervisor and advise her that Nurse X is giving an incorrect image of both childbirth and the hospital. This nurse appears to view childbirth as a demeaning process, undeserving of dignity. Her attitude — and that of the anesthetist — can only serve to damage the positive conditioning process of Prepared Childbirth. It's an attitude that all too often results in the kind of painful, traumatic birth she predicts — a kind of negative wish fulfilment!

Similarly, when Nadia A. arrived at a large general hospital recently her confidence in Prepared Childbirth was undermined in the first twenty minutes. "The admitting nurse's attitude was upsetting. Aside from a brusque, unsupportive attitude, she told me that I was too 'hyper' for natural childbirth, I'd be in pain and should have an epidural.''

Beverley S. encountered the same nurse and found her treatment equally disconcerting. "I know that not all nurses are familiar with the techniques we were using," she told me, "And I'm sure that many women who are not prepared ask for 'natural childbirth' and eventually need an epidural, but that's not the point. I feel that the woman's choice should be respected. Instead of talking down to us, we'd feel much more confident if she said something like, 'That's a good decision', or even 'Good luck!' or even nothing at all!''

Admission procedures frequently do nothing to support the couple's self esteem. Freda D. had discussed with her doctor the possibility of having a clip at home rather than a full shave. It was her second child and she decided clipping was preferable. Her doctor agreed. But the nurse was unsupportive. "It was such a little thing, really. I told the nurse that the doctor agreed, but she insisted because all women had shaves and I didn't want an infection, did I?''

Beverley also had her doctor's permission to bypass the shave. "The nurse was horrified and said 'At this hospital all women have shaves!' I stuck to my guns and didn't have a shave, but when it came time for delivery, one nurse yelled, "She's not ready!" This was almost funny — the baby's head was right there. Fortunately the doctor arrived and confirmed that I was 'ready'; Josh agreed and was born minutes later. That nurse humiliated me — quite unnecessarily, I'm sure.''

Shaving may be a small issue, but Beverley's experience illustrates a prevalent staff attitude guaranteed to lower a couple's self-esteem. Inadvertently, nurses, interns and residents can sabotage many weeks of training by disparaging the efforts of the woman or her coach. Plantevin writes, "Even if they (the staff) themselves do not believe in the value of psychoprophylactic methods for pain relief, they must not by their attitude discourage the patient or destroy her faith in the method she has chosen.''[1]

Ada C. was unfortunate enough to encounter such a resident. "I explained to the resident what I was doing and he said condescendingly, 'Oh yes, the Lamaze Method — isn't that a form of birth control?' Then he told me that he thought it stupid to bother with the techniques because most women needed an epidural anyway. I felt as though we'd been foolish to do all that training — and that it couldn't possibly work.''

Elaine B. encountered a similar attitude in a resident, coupled with what she felt was unnecessary roughness. So she complained to the head nurse. ''It was my second baby and I knew internals didn't have to be painful. Every time the resident came in he just ignored me — never asked how I was getting along, didn't even introduce himself. I asked him to be more gentle and he looked at me as though I were nothing. I felt terribly humiliated.''

Inadequate explanations for hospital procedures are responsible for a great deal of worry and anxiety. For example, Ann H. recently experienced birth in a way she later described as depressing.

> *The resident decided to install an internal fetal heart monitor. As far as I know it was his decision, not my doctor's. Its installation was uncomfortable. I'm not questioning the medical management of my labor, but nobody bothered to explain to me why the monitor was necessary. I was worried that something was wrong, and particularly with what I found to be an uncomfortable procedure . . .*

Marnie A. encountered a similar set of circumstances which, she feels, undermined ''birth with dignity'' for her as well as creating needless anxiety:

> *I'd been induced because of high blood pressure — that was O.K. as my doctor had explained it carefully. My husband had helped me through hours of very long, strong, erratic contractions — we'd been prepared for that — but toward the end a resident came in and poked around, then she called a nurse and yelled, "God — she's*

a breech!!" And she left. We'd gone over breech in classes and I knew it could be straightforward or complicated. But I was terrified that this was a terrible breech and my baby was going to die. Fortunately, my doctor arrived: he assured me that the baby was not in breech positon and that everything was perfectly normal — but that resident sure needs more information on dealing with women in labor!

The choice of birth position in one which frequently causes unnecessary discomfort. As discussed in Chapter 3, the lithotomy position is not only uncomfortable but physiologically undesirable for birth. But many hospitals still require all women to give birth while lying flat on their backs.

The use of stirrups normally increases the need for episiotomy, by increasing the tension on the muscles and increasing the chances of tearing. Many women who wish to avoid unnecessary episiotomies request that stirrups not be used. But many doctors react to this request with frowns of disapproval.

I discussed the possibility of avoiding episiotomy with my doctor, who did them routinely. I asked if I could avoid stirrups, as I had in England for the birth of my first child, where episiotomy wasn't thought necessary. He told me flatly that his patients all used stirrups, but if I didn't want episiotomy maybe he could avoid it . . .

When the time came the staff insisted on stirrups and I felt I was being hurried along with the pushing. I could almost see the doctor checking his watch. He didn't give me any instructions which are necessary to avoid tearing, I've read. He just stood there and let me tear. His attitude was, "Well, I gave you what you asked for" . . .

—Kaye G.

I recently discussed episiotomy with a young, otherwise charming doctor, who was speaking at a workshop of physiotherapists and nurses. "I don't see why you give it so much importance," he said, "It's just a little incision and there's nothing to it." Most of the women present were mothers and they all disagreed quite loudly. Most of them had memories of uncomfortable stitching, sore perineums for days afterwards and being unable to sit properly for up to a week. Just a little incision? Perhaps his view would change if he were faced with "just a little incision routinely made in the scrotum!"

"No one ever asks women about what they want," says Reva, "It seems to me that every woman I'vs talked to has a bad memory about episiotomy. Sure we all agree that if it's necessary, go ahead. But I've read about what's done in other countries and I have a friend who gave birth in England three times and never needed episiotomy. If it's not always necessary but just done so that the doctor can get back to his office quickly, that's a pretty sad situation."

Often couples ask for more pillows for delivery or perhaps to have the head of the table tilted a little. Outrageous?

> We were treated like freaks, because we asked if I could avoid stirrups and have an extra pillow with the table tilted a little. I know these tables can't be tilted much because they're all in one piece and the woman will slip, but a little seemed possible. The nurse told me, "The normal position is good enough for most women!" It was a complete put-down and I was so upset I didn't say another word.
>
> —Sheila B.

Many women have a claustrophobic fear of the handcuffs used routinely in most hospitals to attach the mother's hands to the handgrips used in pushing. Introduced when general anesthesia was in vogue, they were supposedly to keep the woman's hands out of the way. But I've never seen a prepared woman out of control during delivery.

The only thing I was adamant about was those hand-cuffs. When I asked the nurse if I could avoid them she told me that they were to stop my hands from slipping when I pushed and the doctor didn't want me reaching and touching the baby. I said I'd rather take my chances with the slipping and I wouldn't touch if he wanted me not to. She glared and put them on — I couldn't do a thing.

—Shirley S.

I have also received many complaints from women who were embarrassed or disturbed by procedures carried out only for teaching purposes:

I gave birth at a big teaching hospital and I seemed to be getting a lot of unnecessary internals by a variety of people. Finally, one man — he never introduced himself — curtly told me he was installing an internal monitor. It was uncomfortable — I don't think he'd ever done one before — and nobody, not even my doctor, ever explained why it was necessary. The birth had absolutely no complication. I think now that I was used as a guinea pig for teaching purposes.

—Faith R.

It's difficult — almost impossible — to achieve childbirth with dignity when you're strapped down against your wishes, or used as an involuntary guinea pig. The taboo against touching the newborn is groundless. More and more hospitals are waiving the "don't touch" rule and allowing the mother to touch her newborn, as is routine in most other countries of the world.

Although breastfeeding on the delivery table is becoming more accepted under pressure of thousands of women, La Leche League and childbirth education groups, it is still far from routine. "When I asked to nurse my baby right away, the doctor said he didn't see why that was necessary," says

Francine. "But she was my baby and if I wanted to nurse her I felt they should have respected this reasonable wish."

The key words in a client-oriented birth experience are *support* and *flexibility* in non-medical matters. Following the birth of their babies, each of the couples in my course completes a detailed "birth report". One section deals with hospital support. These following quotes are samples of recent births:

> *During delivery, the doctor sat with an intern, and they muttered constantly. He was using me to explain techniques . . . but he didn't inform me of progress at all. Finally the baby was dumped on my tummy . . . After the doctor let the intern stitch me up, he went back to his paperwork without a single remark to me.*
> —*Renee S.*

> *. . . ranged from helpful to extremely annoying . . .*
> —*Heather R.*

> *Case room staff kept urging me to have an epidural . . . not a pleasant experience.*
> —*Teresa C.*

True Client-Oriented Births

Fortunately, many of my couples manage to get client-oriented childbirth, thanks to their hard work, communication and the many warm, compassionate staff members in our labor rooms. Each week the comments on the hospital staffs become more enthusiastic. One truly client-oriented birth was Barbara and Michael's:

> *We had read Leboyer's book, **Birth Without Violence**, and it made a lot of sense to us. Our doctor read the book and we discussed the ins and outs of it thoroughly. When the time came the doctor left a dinner party to be there. As pre-arranged, although far from routine at the hospital, we remained in a labor room*

throughout the entire birth. I didn't require medication and I'd given myself a clip so the shave was avoided. Michael is a painter and he'd brought some of his paintings into the room to make it more homey.

I delivered lying on my side to minimize the chance of tearing. Michael didn't leave the room once. The lights were dimmed for the birth and the baby given to me immediately to nurse. The doctor waited until the cord blood stopped pulsating, a full six minutes. Then Michael, who had brought a plastic bath in, went to fill it and the nurses gave him sterile water at the right temperature. He held our son in the water and the baby relaxed immediately.

We had him with us for an hour or so. Michael crouched in a corner holding the baby, crooning to him, while the baby gazed at him. The doctor and staff couldn't have been more supportive or enthusiastic. I think they enjoyed it!

The birth of our daughter Tilke was a truly client-oriented, dignified and wonderful experience. Although it was at the hospital where I had taught for six years, it needed considerable discussion and preparation to have what we had chosen. Labor moved quickly — so quickly that I arrived at the hospital fully dilated and walked into the delivery room. No one complained about the purple socks which I wore throughout to keep my feet warm.

As previously arranged, I was accompanied by a midwife who worked in the case room, British trained and a dear friend. The doctor arrived and stood by while she attended the birth. I'd chosen to avoid stirrups so the bed remained intact. I tried side-lying several times — no one batted an eyelid. As the head crowned, Sally applied counter pressure to the perineum. As it happened I did tear — slightly — but it gave me little discomfort and it was my choice.

As labor had moved so quickly, there had been no shave or enema. David and I will always remember that moment as a lovely intimate one.

In order for childbirth to be given the dignity it deserves, childbirth education is a must to reduce fear and thereby pain and equip the woman with understanding of her body and "tools" with which to work with labor. Rarely is unprepared childbirth in our culture a positive experience. In the Introduction to this book, nursing instructor in obstetrics, Georgiana Kish writes of her first unprepared birth — an experience she will always regret. Happily, her memory of the birth of her second child was the joyous event of which she had been deprived the first time.

> *The nurse cheerfully asked whether we would like tea or coffee as I was only 3 cms dilated. We were soon laughing over names and were in excellent spirits.*
>
> *The nurse came in frequently to check the heart rate. She was an advocate of Prepared Childbirth and wished more women would attend classes.*
>
> *Labor progressed. I was working hard with breathing techniques. Between contractions we were still joking.*
>
> *The contractions grew hard but the whole process seemed so much more fun than the last time. Suddenly I felt the urge to push.*
>
> *I dimly heard instructions to push.*
>
> *I yelled for my glasses. Then three good pushes and "It's a boy!"*
>
> *I felt as I have never felt in my life. Exhilarated, joyous, free of pain. Albert and I were ecstatic!*

Not every woman wants to sidestep routines, avoid stirrups or do anything other than have her baby comfortably. But for true childbirth with dignity, fear and pain must be minimized, full support for whatever the woman is doing must be given and nothing must be done to damage the couple's self-esteem.

Birth With Complications

In 1975, I watched the birth of a baby with a cleft palate in Amsterdam. I had watched a similar North American birth a few years earlier which had proven traumatic for all concerned.

The baby had been born, with both parents present. Without a word, the father was ordered to leave, the mother was given general anesthesia without a word of explanation. Neither parent saw the baby for twenty-four hours after birth. When the mother was brought her baby she didn't want to look because she was terrified the child was hideously deformed. She left hospital depressed and not wanting to discuss the child. Not a thought had been given to the parents' dignity or self-esteem in this matter and considerable pain had been caused.

In contrast, as the Dutch baby emerged and we saw the cleft palate, the doctor placed a piece of sterile gauze over the lower half of the face and held it up to the parents. "Here is your baby. Touch him. He is beautiful but he has a problem with his palate. In twenty-four hours we can put a plate in the roof of the mouth and at four months we can correct the rest."

The parents touched the child. I left, close to tears. When I returned they were cuddling their son and the gauze was removed. "He is beautiful", the mother told him, "We love him!" Truly birth with dignity.

In complicated labors, the need for dignity is most apparent, particularly if possible complications are diagnosed well before the actual birth. But I've received countless phone calls from women who are upset because of inadequate explanations. "My doctor told me that at his hospital, they're doing mostly Caesareans for breech births. He told me that my baby is breech and refused to give me any more information . . ." one typical client told me. In such cases, much anxiety could be eliminated by treating both parents as mature adults who deserve adequate explanations and a right to participate in decision-making. Few women would deny the need for Caesarean in a true complication, but many breech births are uncomplicated. My client was prepared to accept her doctor's decision if complications were likely, but "He didn't even tell me exactly what position the baby was in and why Caesarean was necessary."

Zendy M. had a similar complaint. Because of fetal distress, her doctor performed a Caesarean, and her son — fortunately fine and healthy — was found to have an unusually short cord. Zendy was thankful for the procedure and felt that medical care was excellent — but she described the anxiety caused by a lack of continuity and little information:

> As a result of some tests, the doctors decided to induce me. I was hooked up to so much equipment that I felt totally helpless. They wouldn't let me phone my husband, and it took ages before anyone would call him . . . When I asked one doctor what was wrong, he told me not to worry my pretty little head . . .
>
> I wanted the facts and was prepared to face the worst — but not knowing, I began to imagine all sorts of terrible things. By the time they were prepping me for a Caesarean — still without any explanation to me or my husband — I was reduced to tears. If only they had treated me as an adult, I could have been more relaxed and helpful . . .

In each of the previous cases, the issue is human dignity — not medical competence. Both women were fully prepared to cooperate with the doctors, but neither was given a chance. In sharp contrast is Anne J.'s Caesarean birth, which she described as follows:

> My baby was presenting foot first and prior to the labor my doctor explained that it might be a complicated delivery. So when Bill and I arrived at the hospital, we had realistic expectations — we were prepared to cope with whatever happened. We had

*discussed epidural with our doctor who thought it was a
wise idea in case of a difficult delivery. My breathing
techniques were going well . . . I was totally in control,
but I agreed with him that epidural was a good idea . . .*

*Before the anesthetist gave me the epidural, he spent
five minutes explaining in detail what he was doing. Bill
was allowed to stay the whole time . . .*

*My doctor arrived, examined me, and told the nurse,
"I feel a foot, it's a high breech, get the O.R. ready."
He explained the need for Caesarean and asked which
incision I'd prefer (bikini or regular) and told me I
could have epidural only, as we had discussed. He
showed the X-Rays to Bill and explained why Caesarean
was necessary . . .*

*Although a nurse had tried to arrange to have Bill
watch the operation from the observation room, the
doctor decided there was not enough staff to have
someone with him. I kissed Bill and went in to have my
baby . . .*

*The anesthetist held my hand and patted my forehead
and talked to me calmly. Then suddenly I had a beautiful baby girl. She was shown to me . . . the doctor took
Bill to the nursery where he was given 30 minutes with
her before joining me . . . We were so impressed with
the staff and the care we received . . .*

I received this letter from Anne, along with a photo of herself — smiling radiantly and holding her daughter — taken by
Bill a few hours after the birth. The photo and letter attest to
the fact that a complicated birth can be untraumatic —
joyful, even — if medical personnel make the little extra
effort to ensure that both mother and father know exactly
what is happening.

Patient's Bill of Rights

The rights to information, and considerate, respectful care
are among those outlined in the Patient's Bill of Rights,

affirmed by the board of trustees of the U.S. American Hospital Association on November 17, 1972. Trustees approved this bill in the hope that it would contribute to more effective patient care, and greater satisfaction to patient, physician and hospital.[2]

The Newsletter of the International Childbirth Education Association comments on the Bill: "No catalogue of rights can guarantee for the patient the kind of treatment he has a right to expect. A hospital has many functions to perform . . . All these activities must be conducted with an overriding concern for the patient, and above all, the recognition of his dignity as a human being."

In Canada, a growing body of lay and professionals is equally concerned with the dignity of the patient. As yet there is no Patient's Bill of Rights, but a bill similar to that of the A.H.A. has been proposed. Recently, Dr. John Marian of Saskatoon, Saskatchewan wrote in a publication for the province's Association on Human Rights:

> *A non-person is created by eliminating individuality, uniqueness, self-disclosure, personal space, individuality of choice, decisions and mobility, and by implementing conformity . . . Incomplete screens, semi-public examination, body indignities such as rectal and vaginal examinations, enemas, all contribute to the invasion of privacy. Doctors or nurses who ask others, in the presence of the patient, how the patient is feeling and doing, reduce the patient to an object.*

Many of the rights listed in the A.H.A. bill are also mentioned by the Canadian Medical Association in its Code of Ethics, the World Medical Association in its International Code of Medical Ethnics, and the Canadian Council on Hospital Accreditation in its guide to hospital accreditation.

Although a Bill of Rights may help to advance the cause of human dignity in hospitals, you should be able to achieve this goal by treating hospital staff like human beings and making it quite clear that you expect the same treatment. Most patient complaints do not question medical management; rather, they deal with communication breakdown. You share the responsibility in this area. If you don't discuss what you'd like, the staff will not be aware of your needs as a human being in childbirth.

How to Get Childbirth with Dignity

1.   Choose your doctor very carefully (see Chapter 5) and discuss with him the details of how the birth will proceed under normal conditions — e.g. not using stirrups if all is normal. Include also a discussion about your doctor's colleague and their basic views. If you wish to be together during admission procedures and internals it helps to clear this with him/her in advance.

2.   Discuss with your doctor his/her views in case of complications. Stress that you'd like to be given all information at the time if there are unexpected complications. Discuss his/her approach to Caesarean births, and whether he allows the father to be present in this situation, if regional anesthetic is used.

3.   When you arrive at the hospital, explain pleasantly and politely to everyone you come in contact with that you're using Prepared Childbirth, assuming that they'll be supportive.

4.   Expect some introduction from people who come into your room during the course of labor. If someone in a white coat strolls in and says, "I wonder would you step outside," to the man and asks the woman to lie down for an internal, you are quite justified in saying, "I'm sorry, I don't think you introduced yourself," or "I don't think we know who you are." As long as you're polite and pleasant, this precaution helps ensure that you're treated as *people*. Sometimes such casual treatment is merely an oversight, but often it's the result of staff thinking of you as "The woman in no. 6".

5.   If tests or high-risk procedures are required, ask for a

brief explanation of the need and outcome. You have a right to this information! If you encounter disturbing information such as Marnie and her husband did, the coach should say, "Listen, we're pretty worried — you sound as though this breech is likely to be a problem. Can you please tell us more?"

6. Suppose at the last moment — after being assured that you can give birth in the position you've chosen — the staff seem desperate to put you in stirrups? In such a situation, the coach can help by saying something along the lines of, "I don't think you understand — we have doctor's permission not to use stirrups and he told us you'd all be very helpful."

7. You have a right to refuse to be a "teaching subject" for medical students, interns, or other obstetrical trainees. Teaching procedures can be carried out pleasantly, and you might not object to them. But if you find yourself subjected to unwarranted procedures — particularly by young men and women who seem to be students — you are within your rights to demand both an introduction and an explanation, and to refuse to be used as a guinea pig, if this seems to be the case.

8. Finally, throughout the hospital experience, both mother and father should try to behave like intelligent, calm and prepared adults, and to presume that staff members will too.

10   The right to family-centered maternity care

After Andrew was born, cuddled, nursed and "confiscated", I was sent to my room — there to be ridiculed for any attempts at adult or independent behaviour. Upon arrival I was greeted by a jug of lemonade and instructions to drink it and make "nice pee pees." Then I asked for my baby. "He'll come soon enough, why don't you just rest and forget him," the nurse told me.

I was obnoxious enough to get him eight hours after birth, but when I asked to have him four hours later, at 2 a.m., all hell broke loose. The head of the nursery came down to tell me that it just wasn't done and that I was tired. I tried to explain that I was fine and could judge my own fatigue, to no avail. I requested "rooming-in" and asked everyone when my baby would be brought. Nobody would tell me.

At 6 a.m. I saw Andrew again. He was now 16 hours old and still not in my room. I showered, dressed and walked to the nursery. They said they would keep him until my pediatrician saw him. I asked if this was "policy" and they

*said no, so I was promised that Andrew would move in at 10
a.m.*

*When my doctor came I mentioned that they were holding
my baby for ransom — and as a result Andrew and his travelling bed soon arrived. I was breastfeeding, a wise decision I
thought — until all my efforts were scoffed at and the sight of
a bare breast resulted in belittling comments like, "Poor baby
is hungry" — "Would you like a bottle for him?" and "You
don't have enough milk for him."*

*I was not a successful breastfeeder with my first child and I
was nervous. I asked a nurse to help at the next feeding. She
didn't appear. Once again I read my breastfeeding book. I
was a real sight, baby in one arm, sucking, and the book in
the other. After two days of this frustration I left.*

— Carol H.

Carol H.'s son is now in primary school and there have
been enormous changes in the way nursing staff regard and
treat new mothers since he was born. Many large hospitals
have changed their policies, thanks to letters like Carol's and
other pressure from consumers. Attitudes toward breastfeeding have altered so significantly that today in some hospitals
the majority of new mothers choose to feed their infants this
way.

Hospitals have shortened observation periods, allow
fathers to visit at any time they wish, and also permit sibling
visits. Some offer these services as a matter of choice; at
others, though, you must ask for them — and do it in a way
that your request will be granted. To get what you want, you
need the facts.

Early Mother-Child Separation

*The human baby should have the advantage of every
other newborn animal. He should seek his mother's
breast and feel his mother's body as soon after birth as
possible and stay there. He should not be taken away to
cry alone in a nursery until someone comes along to give*

*routine care while his mother waits hungrily for him
down the hall.*

> —*Dr. Morris Gold, quoting his
> wife, an obstetrical nurse.*

Medical textbooks describe the first twelve hours after birth as a critical period, requiring constant observation of both mother and baby. The mother must be checked regularly for general condition, to make sure that bleeding is normal and that the uterus is shrinking. The baby's condition — color, temperature, respiration — must be watched. In most North American hospitals, the mother is observed in a "recovery" area while her baby goes to a central nursery where it is given a bottle of glucose and water.

Few would argue with the need for observation. However, in most countries outside North America, observation is performed without separating mother and baby. On this continent, a growing number of obstetrical units, aware of the importance of mother/baby contact, have made efforts to meet family needs by giving mother, father and baby up to half an hour together after the birth. But still at many hospitals, contact is restricted to a token cuddle before taking the baby to the central nursery. Yet a large number of research studies indicate that the first hours after birth are vital to successful mother-child imprinting and bonding.

Experiments with goats, cows and sheep demonstrate that separation of mother and baby for a period as short as one to four hours may result in disturbed mothering patterns, such as failure of the mother to care for her young, butting it away and feeding her own and other offspring indiscriminately. Renowned child psychologist Lee Salk writes, "If as little as one hour goes by after a sheep gives birth and if the mother sheep does not have the opportunity during that time to nuzzle or lick the lamb, the sheep's attachment to the lamb is significantly weakened. As a result, her offspring may be unable to develop normally because of the weakened offspring-parent bond."[1]

Salk believes that weakening of the human mother-baby relationship may be similarly affected. His studies show that the tendency of new mothers is to hold their babies over their hearts, regardless of right or left handedness. Where there is prolonged separation, mothers tend to hold the baby on the right side more frequently.

In the early 1970's a study team — pediatricians Klaus and Kennell, and psycholinguist Norma Ringler — observed a group of babies at Case Western Reserve Hospital in Cleveland. Children and their mothers were tested at birth — and followed up to the age of five years.

Studies by Klaus and Kennell on human behaviour at birth reinforce Salk's work. To determine whether current hospital practices affect later maternal behaviour, they divided 28 mothers of similar backgrounds, with full-term babies of similar characteristics, into two groups. One group was given 16 more hours of mother-baby contact in the first three days of life than the control group who received standard hospital treatment for mother and baby. Maternal behaviour was measured at one month using a standard interview, an examination of the baby and a filmed feeding. Extended-contact mothers showed increased reluctance to leave their babies with someone else, usually stood and watched during the examination, showed greater soothing behaviour and engaged in significantly more fondling and eye-to-eye contact than mothers in the control group. Follow-up assessment at one year showed similar results — healthier maternal behaviour in the group that received more initial mother-baby contact.[2]

The most extreme result of impaired mothering due to separation may be the battered child syndrome. Klaus believes that early separation may indeed be a factor. He writes, "The formation of close emotional ties may remain permanently incomplete if extended separation occurs."

Extended mother-baby contact in the first three days of life may even have a dramatic positive effect on your child's intelligence. In 1976, Dr. Norma Ringler, psycholinguist on the Cleveland team, showed long range effects of the first 72 hours of life. When the children were two years old, an analysis of speech patterns showed that mothers given extended contact with their babies used more questions, more informative speech and in general talked more to their children than mothers in the control group. "Asking a question shows the mother sees the child as someone separate, because she expects a response," explained Ringler. At five years the extended-contact group scored consistently higher on intelligence tests than children in the control group, with better comprehension, advanced vocabulary and expressive ability. Ringler attributes the differences to a special feeling between mother and child fostered by extended contact in the first days of life. She agrees with Kennell that a "baby's ultimate development may be greatly influenced by early and extended contact. Those who care for mothers and infants should be aware of the possible long term effects — both positive and negative — of the early post partum period." [3]

One of the factors influencing many couples to seek home birth rather than the safety of a hospital is the observation period. Founder of the Washington group Home Oriented Maternity Experience (HOME) geared to making home birth a safe as well as satisfying alternative, Pilar Farnsworth gave birth to her last three children at home for this reason. She believes that separation of mother and child at birth are damaging to human nature:

> *Children in America are placed in lonely glass cribs under bright lights away from their mothers for a period of six or twelve or twenty four hours. The "Observation Period" exemplifies to perfection modern man's alienation from nature and self . . . In the immediate hours following birth a deep process of binding love happens between mother and child . . . The mother needs to hold her child. She will look, stroke, caress — the unconscious biological intent of this caress is to erase the tension that might exist in this tiny head that*

*has just emerged. She might offer the nipple and the
baby might suck . . . When this immediate need of contact between mother and child after birth is impaired,
rejection mechanisms start to operate. Birth is the first
interaction between a child and the world. It must be an
act of love for the mother and everyone else. It must not
be marred by pain or fear or separation.*[4]

I have been with hundreds of mothers and fathers who
longed to cuddle and meet their babies in a leisurely way at
birth. Too often this is a rushed and awkward moment in the
bustle of a delivery room, the mother unable to make herself
comfortable on the delivery table under the scrutiny of the
well-meaning staff. Too often the father is denied an opportunity to hold his baby because of the rush of the moment.
Very little has been written of father-child bonding, but I
believe that the beneficial effects of fondling and eye-to-eye
contact between father and child are as significant and long
reaching as mother-child contact — one of the more important factors in strengthening the family and providing the
baby with a loving home in which to grow. I have also
watched families relax alone in the recovery cubicle after the
birth — thirty minutes which make a big difference to the
mother, father and baby who get to know each other at their
own pace.

Following birth, few women feel like sleep. This is particularly true for the prepared mother who has had little or no
medication. The hours after birth are a joyous peak of
emotion. At this time, most women have a strong physical
and mental need for their babies. After the birth of my own
daughter I cuddled and nursed her in the delivery room then
watched as she was carried off to the nursery. After my
husband left, I felt terribly lonely and not at all tired. The
only thing I really wanted was my baby!

One of the excuses for separation is that of the baby's temperature. A heated glass crib is deemed better to keep the
baby warm than its mother's arms. This belief dates back to

the general anesthesia era. Following heavy maternal medication, the temperature of many babies suddenly dropped in the hour or so after birth, and observation was vital. Nor was the mother in any condition to mother. The era of twilight sleep has passed but the physical set-up of the North American maternity unit has not changed. Yet, as I pointed out in Chapter 1, observation of mother and baby in a central area at birth and the following hours is done with little difficulty on the part of the staff in countries such as France and Holland. There, the baby is checked by a pediatrician and — because the majority of women are prepared for birth and require no medication — there is little danger of problems several hours later. In North America, however, the medicated birth is the norm: most staff members are not familiar with wide-awake mothers and babies whose natural instinct is to be together.

Valerie Poulard recently gave birth in the gentle non-violent delivery advocated by Leboyer. She required no medication and says:

> The baby was wide awake and very calm right after birth and I felt wonderful. I nursed my son immediately and he sucked strongly for ten minutes. But then the nurse took him to the nursery. My husband followed . . . he wanted to bring him back to me as soon as he had been checked. During his admission to the nursery, our son really cried for the first time. He lay in his crib wide-awake, and the nurse told my husband that he was an "irritable" baby because he should have been sleeping. It seems the nursery staff so rarely see non-medicated babies that they figured something was wrong!

I spent an afternoon and evening at Amsterdam's large rambling old Wilhemina Gasthuis, an obstetrical unit comparable in size to most North American city units. I have described the births I watched, in Chapter 1 — calm, dignified and with minimum interference. The Dutch believe that newborn humans belong with their mothers, and the medicated baby is rarely a problem — under 5% of Dutch women require medication in labor.

The labor-deliver-recovery cubicles are small and face a central area. In the centre of this area is a table with small "cribs", more like boxes, built into the top. There are nine cribs to the table and lights overhead. Following birth and the initial cuddling, the baby is placed here, in full view of the parents and checked immediately by the pediatrician. He or she is then returned to the parents who stay together in the next hours under the eye of a nurse, whose office area is on one side of the room. No glucose and water is given. Because only 2% of the mothers here need medication, almost without exception the babies are pink and alert and suck vigorously. The value of early breastfeeding is taken for granted. After the initial hours, mother and baby go to their room, the baby in a portable crib at the side of the mother's bed.

At this hospital the baby stays at the bedside but can be sent to a central nursery at night. This is the procedure in France also, where a combination labor-delivery and recovery room makes this simple.

At the Academic (University) Hospital of Amsterdam I saw an ideal. All rooms here contain three beds and adjoin a glass-walled nursery. Babies can either stay with the mother or be wheeled into the little nursery, if she chooses, still within her full view. A nurse cares for the unit as a whole and all baby care is done at the mother's bedside. The mother is free to nurse her child as she deems necessary. Such a system is simple: why is it so rare in North America?

Breastfed: best fed?

Way back in 1923, Mabel Liddiard wrote in "The Mothercraft Manual":

> *Nature has evolved a wonderful plan whereby the stomach is slowly educated to digest normal food. For*

> *the first few days there is found in the breasts a thin
> watery-looking fluid called* **colostrum,** *a most valuable
> food containing a large percentage of protein of the
> same nature as that found in actual blood. Thus it can
> be absorbed into the blood stream with practically no
> effort on the part of the stomach and digestive juices.
> During the first days, this fluid is gradually changed to
> true milk, in which time the baby's stomach and
> digestive juices have been learning how to work ef-
> ficiently. Also the chemical composition of this fluid is
> the same as that with which the baby was fed before
> birth, both having been derived from the mother's
> blood . . . Picture the difference when, a few hours or
> days after birth an entirely strange milk is passed into
> the delicate little stomach.*[5]

"An entirely strange milk" or substance is what most babies receive in the first 24 hours after birth. Recently Halifax pediatrician Dr. Richard Goldbloom deplored the fact the only 15% of Canadian mothers breastfeed their babies.[6] Even if the mother chooses to nurse, sup-plementation of "glucose water" or formula is frequently urged or made routine by hospital "policy".

In 1930, a publication on prenatal care put out by the United States Department of Labor, Children's Bureau, wrote, "It is the first duty of every mother to nurse her baby. Every doctor, nurse or other attendant should insist that the mother nurse her baby and should do everything possible to start the secretion of milk, to promote it, or even bring it back if for any reason it has stopped."[7]

By the end of the nineteen twenties, artificial feeding was a rival to breastfeeding, although the majority of women still nursed. As a result of the promotion of formula by com-mercial companies as "easier, more convenient and nutritious", together with an increase in the number of women wishing to pursue careers outside the house, the bottle replaced the breast for most North American babies.

Currently, many women are returning to breastfeeding. In some hospitals about 40% of women nurse, but across the continent Dr. Goldbloom's estimate of 15% is probably fairly accurate. When I was growing up in Australia, I became accustomed to the slogan "Breastfed is best fed" passed out at baby health centres. In department stores there was a mother's feeding room and breastfeeding was regarded as normal. That was in the sixties. I have been home regularly every two years since 1967: each time I talk with staff at the centres, I am told that fewer women are nursing. Much of the cause rests with inadequate information given by doctors on breastfeeding, commercial promotion of formula feeding and a growing general cultural negativity towards breastfeeding—the bottle has become synonymous with "progress."

In many areas of North America, nursing continues to be regarded as "old fashioned": many obstetricians asked for their views on breastfeeding will say that there's no difference between breast and bottle feeding and why bother nursing? It is true that beautiful, healthy babies can be raised on breast or bottle, and formula can provide adequate nutrition. But there are unique benefits in breastfeeding—and few women are given the facts. My discussions with women in my classes lead me to believe that many wish to nurse but decide not to, because they are afraid they won't "succeed" or because they simply don't have enough information. Instead, they possess a wealth of misinformation—often readily passed on by well intentioned friends.

Some time ago, when I was discussing breastfeeding in class, one of the fathers, a farmer, stressed what is taken for granted in animal husbandry—the importance of "species specific" (e.g., cow's milk for calves, mare's milk for foals) milk for the young animal. And a vast body of research confirms that the benefits of a substance species specific benefits the young human equally.

One big benefit of breastmilk is in the prevention of disease. Pediatrician J.W. Gerrard writes, "Colostrum and breastmilk provide a two pronged attack against pathogenic (disease producing) organisms: a low pH medium which prevents growth of pathogenic E. Coli and immunoglobulins which fight infection. Cow's milk and other foods cause a high pH in the gut where pathogenic organisms thrive, and provide no immunoglobulins with which to fight disease.'' He adds that babies cannot manufacture antibodies against many diseases until they are 9-12 months old: they therefore are totally dependent on antibodies acquired via the placenta and later in colostrum and breastmilk. Gerrard concludes, "Breast milk alone for the first six months provides the best protection."[8]

Doris Haire, in *The Cultural Warping Of Childbirth* cites a study of more than 3,000 children living in a housing project in England (post-penicillin) which showed that the death rate was nine times greater among children who were artificially fed from birth. All the children received the same health team, "Yet among those children who were breastfed there was significantly less incidence of common colds, bronchitis, pneumonia, eczema, asthma, hayfever, colic, gastroenteritis, otitis media, mastoid, whooping cough, measles, german measles and scarlet fever." She goes on to add that colostrum contains antibodies against "Three strains of polio, Coxsackie B virus, two types of colon bacilli which can cause fatal infant diarrhea, pathogenic strains of E coli, and gran negative infections."[9]

In underdeveloped countries, breastfeeding may be a matter of life or death. Recently the World Health Organization deplored the fashion toward bottle feeding in these countries, particularly South America with its questionable water supplies and alarmingly high incidence of disease of infancy, often fatal. Because standards of hygiene are so much better in Canada and the U.S., the bottle is usually as safe as the breast—but the disease prevention factor is relevant anywhere, particularly so if you plan to travel with a young baby.

The breastfed baby is far less likely to develop obesity than the bottle fed infant. Writing in the British Medical Journal, *Lancet,* Dr. B. Hall suggests that breastfeeding has a built-in appetite control. He hypothesizes that the watery milk occurring normally at the beginning of a breastfeeding satisfies the baby's thirst, the higher caloric milk coming toward the end of the feeding. He believes that cow's milk formulae with constant high solute levels do not satisfy thirst. The thirst may be misinterpreted as hunger and the bottle fed baby may be overfed and become obese. He adds that in 1971 in Sheffield, England, 60% of bottle fed babies had weight gains above the 90th percentile; compared to 19% of breastfed babies.

Another theory on the higher incidence of obesity in bottle fed babies is the increased need for sucking which some babies demonstrate. With breastfeeding, additional sucking at the end of a feeding provides a thin stream of milk. With bottle feeding the baby's sucking may be interpreted as hunger and another bottle given.[10]

Cow's Milk an Allergen?

In 1964, at a New York University Conference, Dr. James Glaser related the increase in infant allergies to abandonment of breastfeeding. Glaser believes that many babies react allergically to the foreign protein of cow's milk. When an allergic reaction appears in infants, cow's milk is the most common offender. Not only are babies exposed to foreign protein, but to extremely high amounts of it. Glaser designed a controlled study to see if dermatitis could be prevented by avoiding cow's milk. Glaser followed 96 infants, all potentially allergic, from birth to at least seven months, some as long as ten years. None were given cow's milk for the first three months of life. 88 of the 96 were fed a commercially available soya milk, 51 received some meat-based formula, three were breastfed. A control group was made of 65 siblings of the experimental group who were fed cow's milk from birth. A second control group of 175 infants with similar family histories of allergies was studied. Skin trouble appeared in 30% of the control group (cow's milk fed); only 7%

in the experimental group had skin problems. Development of major allergic disease occurred in 60% of the control group and only 15% in the experimental group.[11]

Sudden Infant Death Syndrome (SIDS) is the name given to a tragic mystery illness which kills a minimum of 25,000 babies each year in the United States and Canada. A seemingly healthy baby is put down to sleep and is discovered by a distraught parent hours later — dead. Death is attributed to unknown cause. Because "unknown disease" cannot be entered on a death certificate it is called heart failure, suffocation or other names. The baby is usually between three weeks and five months old. Post mortem results do not reveal cause of death. In the summer of 1963, so many "crib deaths" occurred that SIDS, often passed over with great secrecy, was publicized. In Philadelphia, 100 SIDS occurred in a single summer week.

In Kentucky, deputy coroner Daniel Stowens, MD of Children's Hospital of Louisville, Kentucky and University of Louisville School of Medicine investigated 2,000 infants who had died of SIDS, in autopsy. Stowens believes SIDS is caused by allergy to cow's milk. Changes he noted included edema — water in the tissues — which appeared uniformly in all the SIDS babies. He noted swelling and pallor of the liver cells without any evidence of metabolic abnormality. He found that urine samples of the dead infants contained the substance nephrosis peptide. He also found changes in the blood vessels of the kidneys. Together, these changes point to a process common in the process of allergy reaction — anaphylactic shock. The body produces antibodies to fight against the protein it cannot absorb — to which it is allergic. These antibodies may produce sudden shock reaction in the system which can result in death.

With an eye to allergy, Stowens discovered that crib deaths did not occur in babies totally breastfed, and rarely in partially breastfed babies. Almost without exception the crib death babies were fed cow's milk formula or cow's milk alone. He believes that some babies do not digest protein from cow's milk, but absorb it whole from the gastrointestinal tract. Sensitization occurs gradually, increasing unobserved until suddenly the body goes into shock — and death results. [12]

I don't want to imply that if you bottle-feed your baby, you are increasing his/her chance of crib death. But I do find it curious that Stowen's findings have received almost no publicity or follow-up. In a matter so devastating as crib death, certainly investigation and follow-up studies to prove or disprove his theory are in order.

More Benefits of Breastfeeding

Believe it or not, breastfeeding can even promote good dental formation in the toothless infant! The most recent Canadian dental study shows that two out of five Canadian children have poor occlusion ("bite") and I have no reason to doubt that the same figures would be true in the U.S. [13] But the many dentists who have participated in my classes as parents-to-be have stressed that the strong sucking necessary in breastfeeding — difficult to duplicate with the bottle — develops correct palate formation and the muscles later used in speech. And research indicates that there is less incidence of orthodontic disproportion and orofacial (jaw) deformities among children who were breastfed. Many bottle babies develop "tongue-thrust" — milk may come too quickly from the bottle and the baby learns to slow the flow with his or her tongue. Resultant tongue-thrust may contribute to later speech problems. [14]

Prolactin, the milk-making hormone, has been shown to increase motherliness and is believed important in maternal attachment. The famous monkey experiments of Dr. Harlow showed increased desire for breastfeeding female monkeys to reach their young than mothers not nursing. Recently, the use of the ergot-derived drugs to accelerate the expulsion of the placenta and prevent bleeding has caused concern to the proponents of breastfeeding. Ergot suppresses the production of prolactin and may in itself provide a handicap to early nursing in the hospital, as well as interfering with the bonding process.[15]

Quite apart from the scientific reasons for breastfeeding, most women I've spoken to quite simply enjoy it. The nursing relationship ensures a warm cuddling with skin to skin contact — it's impossible to prop a baby at the breast! The hormonal reactions of breastfeeding have a relaxing effect on the mother and for the "lazy" woman night feeding is simpler if you're breastfeeding.

Travelling is simple and someone figured that the money saved in breastfeeding in one year would buy a major appliance. Critics argue that it costs that to feed the mother. Good nutrition is necessary, but dramatic changes to a good diet are not necessary. Breastfeeding, moreover, contracts the mother's uterus to normal rapidly and is a natural way of losing weight gained in pregnancy.

Unfortunately, many of the women I've spoken to have run into problems in the first weeks in hospital — usually the result of nonsupportive hospital care and half-hearted counselling from their doctors.

Culture Versus the Breast

At once or in a few weeks, most American mothers reject their own bodies as a source of food for their children, and in accepting the mechanical perfection of a bottle, reaffirm to themselves, and in the way they handle their babies, that the baby too will be much better, the more it learns to use the beautifully mechanical bottle . . . For the primary learning experience that is the physical prototype of the sex relationship — a complementary relation between the body of the mother and the body of the child — is substituted a relationship between the child and an object . . . She is not giving the child herself; she is faithfully, efficiently providing the child with a bottle, external to both of them, sub-

stituting for a direct relationship a relationship mediated by an object.

—Margaret Mead[16]

The neglect of the nursing mother begins in pregnancy. In my own survey of Montreal hospitals, hospitals with the highest incidence of nursing mothers rated 30-40% and those with the lowest 10-12%. This is partly the fault of our culture, but the obstetrician does little to encourage nursing.

> *I asked my doctor if he thought I should breastfeed. He said that it doesn't really matter, bottle feeding is just as good. "Not every woman is cut out for breast-feeding," he finished. I'd read that the baby gets resistance to disease and I had a friend who went to meetings of the breastfeeding group, La Leche League. She told me that it was good for the baby and I would enjoy it, but after my doctor's discouraging comments I didn't even try to nurse. I went to a La Leche meeting with my friend after my baby was born — several months later, to see what it was all about, and I wish I'd tried. If I have another baby I'll certainly nurse."*
>
> *— Amy R.*

Amy's experience is far too common. Doctors rarely give information about breastfeeding and many actively discourage it as "old fashioned". Even if the doctor is in favor of nursing, he or she will probably warn the woman not to be upset if she can't nurse, and assure her that bottle feeding is "just as good". It's a similar misguided — and potentially discouraging — attitude which causes the nurse to caution the laboring woman, "Don't feel guilty if you need an epidural — most women do and you can still have natural childbirth."

In my experience, the decision to breast or bottle feed is often influenced by the attitude of the child's father. Some men — and some women — feel uneasy with the idea of the breast as utilitarian rather than the purely sexual one so often promoted by our culture. (Possibly one can speculate on whether the male infant, deprived of the breast, later turns into a "breast man." Perhaps the word "lecherous" is derived from the Latin *leche* — meaning milk.) However, when women in my classes have discussed feelings about breastfeeding, the reasons for not wanting to are usually: "I don't think I'd have enough milk" . . . "My doctor says I'm too tense" . . . "I've spoken to friends who tried and gave up and I'd rather not try if that's going to happen" . . . "I'm going back to work six weeks after the baby's born and I couldn't nurse then."

The cases where breastfeeding is not possible are few. In fact I can think of only two medical reasons for not breastfeeding: if the baby is born with a cleft palate or if the mother has active tuberculosis — both highly unlikely. Returning to work need not necessarily cancel out breastfeeding. Many women combine breast with bottle feeding to the satisfaction of all concerned. I returned to teaching couples after my child was born and because of flexible hours managed to combine mostly breastfeeding with an occasional bottle with everyone happy. There are cases where a nine to five job resumed very soon after birth makes breastfeeding a difficult choice: bottle feeding may certainly work better but the fact of returning to work doesn't always make nursing impossible.

In a society which regards bottle feeding as the norm, there is little or no opportunity to see a nursing baby and an attitude of distaste is common among many otherwise enlightened people. If you feel uneasy, it's important to examine your feelings. A woman trying unhappily to breastfeed would enjoy her baby and be able to cuddle and relax more easily with a bottle. Many authorities believe that *how* the baby is fed is as important as *what* it is fed within normal limits. But if you feel that you'd like to breastfeed but you're not sure how, it's important to start reading about breastfeeding and get as much accurate information as possible on the subject well beforehand.

If you've decided to breastfeed, choose your hospital wisely. Too often, successful nursing is sabotaged in the hospital by unsupportive staff and by rigid feeding schedules based on the needs of the bottle fed baby — rather than those of the breastfed infant.

Diana phoned me the day after she gave birth. She had been exhilarated following the birth of her vigorous eight pound son. I had spoken to her a few hours after the birth and wondered what had caused her to be so upset. "It's the breastfeeding — I wasn't brought my baby for twenty four hours — that's the routine here and they've been giving him bottles in the nursery and he won't seem to take the breast. I tried to feed him but it didn't work and they took him back to the nursery and said they'd give him a bottle. That's routine too. I'm afraid that I'm not going to be able to nurse at all!"

Diana was right in the middle of the all too frequent dilemma of breastfeeding versus hospital routines. The baby is born with a strong sucking reflex ("rooting reflex"). If the baby is put to the breast immediately at birth, not only does she receive colostrum and stimulate lactation — but the hormones released quickly shrink the mother's uterus back to normal.

But if the first feeding is withheld until several hours after birth, breastfeeding is handicapped. Frequent sucking ensures a good milk supply and also helps prevent painful "engorgement" — a side-effect of our rigid maternity system, regarded as "normal" by most hospitals:

> *I woke up on the third day and my breasts were huge and hard. I really needed my baby. I didn't get her till much later. When she did come, she'd been given a bottle and didn't suck hard. She was taken back half an hour later. I tried to hand express but I was clumsy and my breasts were getting unbearably painful. When the baby was brought out next time, my breast was so swollen she could hardly get the nipple. If I hadn't been*

determined to nurse I would have given up. As soon as
we got home I nursed her as often as she seemed to want
and it's been going well since then."

— Betty E.

If you want a good start to breastfeeding, make every
effort to nurse your baby immediately after birth. You must
usually obtain "permission" from your doctor to do so — so
make sure that you discuss this question with him/her early in
your pregnancy. And be warned: if my clients' doctors are a
representative sample, you may have to do an excellent job of
communicating what you want, and why it's a good idea.
Among my clients in a recent class, only one couple reported
a doctor who had real enthusiasm for immediate post partum
nursing, and seemed aware of its benefits. Two reported
doctors who said "No problem" — possibly with a few
reservations. But the remaining five doctors seemed horrified
at the question, and gave the following replies:

I'm sorry, but that's not allowed. We're proud of our
neonatal death rate at this hospital and we don't want to
take any chances.

The hospital doesn't have facilities . . .

You'd be pretty upset if your baby choked!

Your baby must be checked at the nursery first. Some
have abnormalities of the digestive system, and we give
every baby a bottle before sending it out to the mother.

The delivery room is too cold . . .

The above doctors would probably be looked on as
misinformed in Western Europe: in each of the ten countries
with the lowest neonatal death rates, nursing immediately
after birth is considered normal and sensible. Unfortunately,
North American doctors' objections are based mainly on
their observation of the babies of heavily medicated mothers

— who have had both analgesia and regional anesthesia during labor.

Such babies usually do not suck as strongly, and — because of mucus and possible temperature fluctuation — need more care than the babies of non-medicated mothers. In the rare case of tracheo-esophageal abnormality which one doctor mentions, Haire suggests that the baby be allowed to nurse under the close observation of nurse and doctor — rather than delaying the feeding until several hours later in the nursery, where professional expertise may not be immediately on hand. In the case of a complicated birth or a baby born with a lot of mucus in nose and mouth, an explanation to the mother, and possible postponement of nursing, would suffice. It's ironic that the doctor who rejected immediate breastfeeding for fear of spoiling neonatal death rate figures works at the same hospital as the doctor who expressed enthusiasm for nursing immediately!

How to Breastfeed Successfully

1. During pregnancy read as much about breastfeeding as you can. *Nursing Your Baby* by Karen Pryor or *The Complete Book Of Breastfeeding* by Wendkos and Olds are a good beginning. In most centres there is a branch of *La Leche League International,* a group of mothers who hold a series of public meetings with deal with all the details you'll want to know about nursing. The League has a medical advisory board and runs a telephone counselling service available to mothers with problems. You'll find the group support excellent and have ample opportunity to watch nursing babies at League meetings. The League puts out its own book, *The Womanly Art Of Breastfeeding.*

2. Ask your doctor well in advance if, all being well with you and your baby, you can nurse immediately after birth. This can be done on the delivery table or in the recovery room (depends on hospital "policy").

3. Choose a hospital which has the shortest possible observation period. The shortest observation period I know of

in North American hospitals is a period of about four hours, following an initial "family time" of about 30 minutes immediately after birth, during which both parents may cuddle their baby. If there is no hospital in your area with an observation period shorter than 24 hours, discuss this situation with your doctor, who may be able to arrange for an exception in your case.

4. If possible, choose a hospital which offers "rooming-in" — meaning that the baby may stay in your room as much (or as little) as you choose. Even if you have been unable to sidestep a long observation period, frequent sucking will bring in a good milk supply. Breast milk is normally digested faster than formula: the four-hour schedule adhered to still by many hospitals often does not suit the needs of the breastfed baby who may cry from hunger three hours after a feeding and be given a bottle if in the nursery. Frequent feedings also avoids painful "engorgement" and sore nipples (sucking is gentler when baby sucks little and often). Many hospitals offer "Complete" or "Modified" rooming in. If you want "Complete" (24 hours a day) you usually need a private room. If you share a room, babies return to the nursery at night. If you do share a room, ask the staff to bring you the baby when she/he wakes at night. If this is not possible ask them to wake you so that you can go to the nursery.

Why Night Feeding?

There are two schools of thought on night feedings. The first is "You'll need your rest — get it now." The second is "It's better to build up a good milk supply before you go home — otherwise you'll be tired from frequent night feedings to build up a good milk supply."

Karen fed her baby at night and recommends it. "I found my breasts would fill and I'd wake up after the first night or so anyway. I got to know Jeremy's night habits that way and there was no dramatic change when I got home."

Joyce slept through the night. "It was nice to rest in the hospital. I had a long difficult labor and I needed the rest, but

I did find that it took a while to get night feedings straightened out at home. Josie had been given a bottle at nights in the hospital and I didn't seem to have enough milk the first few nights home, so I was up every couple of hours in the night, and I didn't feel too happy about that.''

Most hospitals offer some sort of rooming-in plan, but this may not begin until after the first day. Ask the doctor if you can have your baby sooner than that. Ask the head nurse. Usually you'll find her sympathetic, and she has the authority to get you wahat you're asking for. If you're at a hospital which is still on a four-hour schedule, speak to the head nurse and see if you can be brought the baby when he or she cries. Usually such hospitals have a far higher incidence of bottle feeding than breast and the nurses may modify routines for you.

Supplementary Bottles?

It is routine at almost every hospital to give one bottle of glucose and water or water during the observation period, to observe sucking and swallowing and to prevent "dehydration". The mother's colostrum serves this purpose, but if mother and baby are separated, the baby does not get the colostrum. Many mothers are worried that their babies become "bottle spoiled". The sucking required for breast is stronger than that for bottle. If supplementary bottles are given, the baby might not suck well at the breast, but suck vigorously at the bottle.

To avoid "bottle spoiling", you can ask your doctor or pediatrician to write on your baby's chart, "No bottles by request." Choosing your pediatrician beforehand gives you an opportunity to discuss hospital feeding procedures in advance. If you choose a pediatrician who is enthusiastic about breastfeeding, he or she will gladly write the request for no bottles on the chart. Unless there are unusual circumstances, this request will probably be followed.

Rose says: "I didn't want bottles given and I simply asked the nurses that no bottles be given. They weren't and I had plenty of milk. The only negative comment was "You're nursing far too long,' but I wasn't having sore nipples and it seemed fine for the baby and me. It's important to prepare your nipples if you want to nurse. I started this at the fifth month of pregnancy and I haven't had any problems."

I've said it before, but I'll repeat it again: preparation ahead of time is your most useful tool for coping with *any* hospital situation!

If You Have Other Children

A "family-centered" hospital should care about the other children in the family. I first became aware of the benefits of sibling visiting when it was introduced some years ago at the Catherine Booth Hospital. At first, some staff objected, on the grounds of the risk of infection and misconduct. But there was no evidence of infection, and the presence of little children several afternoons a week added a lively atmosphere which most would not refer to as misconduct! I never saw any problems resulting from the practice and it is slowly coming into other city hospitals. Dr. Lee Salk, child psychologist, makes much the same observation in "Preparing For Parenthood":

> *Not once did I observe anything that was psychologically upsetting to the child. In fact, I remarked upon the opposite. The little children were delighted to see their mothers and the mothers took great pleasure in showing the new babies to their older children. Since sibling visiting is important to your child's emotional health I sincerely hope that hospitals will modify the antiquated procedures which now keep little children away from the maternity wards.*[16]

One objection to sibling visitation is the fact that the children cry when it is time to go. Dr. Salk believes it healthier to have a number of small separations than one prolonged separation, despite the tears.

Father Visiting

"We do not regard the father as a visitor" is the policy of several of the family-centred hospitals, but unfortunately not all hospitals agree. Many centers still restrict the father to "visiting hours" of an hour or so each day. Fathers from my classes agree that having the opportunity to visit whenever they wished made it easier to support their mates and share baby care. I am a great believer in the need for Paternity Leave: for the father restricted to an hour or so of visiting, baby care is usually restricted to a few cuddles. If the father may come at any time, he can attend baby bath care demonstration, change the baby and take an active part in learning how to care for his child.

"It was great — I'd changed Emily in the hospital, and my wife had asked if a nurse could watch while we did her bath. So that when they came home I could share from the start. I think the man would really feel left out if he couldn't help," says Eric S.

His wife agrees and adds, "It took a lot of the strain of responsibility off me. I knew that if I wanted 'time out', Eric could take over. I have a lot of friends who got depressed because their husbands didn't share the baby much. That's not going to happen with us. It's more fun this way."

In short, "family-centered" care takes into consideration the needs of each family member involved in the arrival of a new baby.

How To Choose Your Hospital

"My doctor was fine," Helen told me, "but that finished at the birth. The hospital didn't encourage breastfeeding. They didn't have rooming-in and every baby was automatically given supplements. I couldn't have the baby for twenty-four hours after birth and then only every four hours. My husband was only allowed to visit for one hour each evening. I'd never have chosen that hospital or that doctor if I'd known more about the hospital he was affiliated with."

Your choice of hospital is limited to the one of your doctor's affiliation. Therefore the choice of doctor should be made according to your choice of hospital. The following steps will help you choose a hospital which will help you assume an active role in the care and responsibility for your child from the moment of birth.

Step One: As soon as you've made an appointment to see a doctor, phone the hospital of his or her affiliation and ask to be fitted into a "hospital tour". All "family centered" hospitals have these tours, usually arranged through the maternity nursing office or physiotherapy department. They are frequently given in the evening for couples. If the hospital offers this service, it's a good sign.

Step Two: If you are looking for a hospital which is truly family-centered, the following list of questions will help you in your selection:

- Are childbirth preparation classes given at the hospital? Are these provided in the evenings? Is the father included? Do many staff members from different departments teach?
- Are staff familiar with prepared childbirth? (Lamaze Method, for example?) Is there any in-service education?
- Do most fathers attend birth?
- Is breastfeeding immediately after birth encouraged?
- How soon after birth is the baby brought to the mother for feeding?
- Is "rooming-in" encouraged? How soon after birth does this start? Is a private room necessary for rooming-in"?
- Does the same nurse care for mother and baby ("mother-baby care")? This provides continuity of care.
- If the mother requests "no supplements" to breastmilk is this wish adhered to under normal conditions?
- Will the mother be brought the baby for night feedings or must she go to the nursery?
- Is there open visiting for fathers?
- Can children under twelve visit?
- Is a baby bath demonstration given — group or privately?
- What percentage of women breastfeed?

Step Three: It is relatively easy to find the answers to these questions during your visit. You have already learned the answers to the first question at your doctor's visit. If classes are given at the hospital, these tend to reflect the attitudes of the obstetrical department. If classes are not provided, the hospital is probably unfamiliar with Prepared Childbirth and possibly lacks many of the elements you want. If the hospital gives day classes only, thus excluding fathers, chances are the staff are not familiar with couple-oriented childbirth. This is not always true, but hospitals which are enthusiastic about family-centered care are usually eager to provide necessary preparation for man and woman. If there are couple-oriented evening classes, you're well on the right track.

If several departments — e.g. physiotherapy, nursing, dietary department and an obstetrician — share in the teaching of the classes, it's a step in the right direction. In a completely couple-oriented and family-centered hospital, all staff usually take some part in preparation. How do you find out if there is in-service education for staff? You might ask, "Do all the nurses watch films of prepared childbirth?" or "I guess all the nurses can help with the Lamaze techniques?" The answer you're given will give you a general idea of the staff's attitude.

If most fathers attend the birth, chances are the staff are familiar with or supportive of Prepared Childbirth. If breastfeeding immediately after birth is encouraged, you can expect a hospital atmosphere which understands the needs of the breastfeeding mother. If you are told it's "not allowed", probably schedules will not be as flexible as you would like. If you are told that it depends on the doctor, ask if many doctors "allow" it. If a few do, but it is not done frequently, ask how many women breastfeed. If it's about 40%, you may get what you'd like. If it's under 25%, this hospital is probably not geared to the breastfeeding mother.

Most family-centered hospitals will bring the baby to the mother four to eight hours after the birth. If it's longer than twelve hours, other policies may not be flexible enough.

Ideally, rooming-in will be provided for in the first 12-18 hours after birth (preferably sooner). There should be similar "rooming-in" if you share a room. If the same nurse cares for mother and baby, there tends to be more continuity of care and the mother-baby are regarded as a unit. This is usually a feature of a family-centred hospital. (Rooming-in does *not* mean "you're on your own!" Nursing care and teaching are still part of the program.)

The hospital you are looking for will not give supplements if you request otherwise. If you are told "All babies are given supplements in the nursery," expect other features which are not in the best interests of mother or baby.

You will find having the baby brought to you far less tiring than walking to the nursery in the middle of the night: if the babies are not brought, usually the majority of women do not make the effort to nurse at night.

Fathers are not regarded as visitors at family-centered hospitals. Sibling visiting is another sign of the flexible hospital for which you are looking. Finally, the hospital should give you and your mate ample opportunity to learn to care for your child, both in group sessions and individually.

Step Four: You have assessed the atmosphere of the hospital, the attitude of the staff and have had most of your questions answered. If you like the general feeling of the obstetrical floor and if on most scores the hospital "passes" you'll feel relieved. If there are some points which make you unhappy, discuss these with your doctor — he might be able to help. Or try to talk with the obstetrical supervisor. In some cases, though, there may be no solution except a compromise — or a change of doctor and hospital. If the hospital includes fathers routinely in birth and the post partum stay, if rooming-in is provided and if you can have your baby in the first eight hours after birth, you've picked a winner!

But even in a fairly good hospital, you may encounter problems with individuals. The following chapter outlines some possible situations, and gives you UPC techniques to deal with most problems you may face.

11 How to get the childbirth you want

Peter and I felt strongly about several things as the birth of our second child approached. I didn't want a routine IV and I wanted to give birth in the labor room if at all possible, without stirrups. When our first child was born two years ago, the IV bothered me. I remember trying desperately to stop myself pushing on the way to the delivery room and the stirrups just weren't comfortable . . .

— Evelyn M.

Appearing as the "guest family" shortly after the birth of their baby daughter, Evelyn and Peter M. told my class how they had used UPC techniques to get the simple childbirth they wanted — in hospital. They had arrived at my classes early in pregnancy. As we discussed birth expectations, Evelyn asked if there were any way of avoiding the routines she had found unpleasant last time. I knew her doctor — an enthusiastic convert to husband-coached childbirth. But although he now welcomed father participation, this doctor was otherwise relatively conservative. Furthermore, he was on staff at the most rigid hospital in the city — the last one in Montreal to include the father at the birth. In this hospital, more than 85% of women in labor receive routine epidurals; IV's on admission are standard policy. Not entirely optimistic about their chances of a labor-room delivery, I nevertheless suggested that Evelyn and Peter discuss with their doctor what they wanted, and why — and that they then tour the hospital and discuss these wishes with the head nurse. This approach worked, Evelyn reported:

> We stressed to the doctor that if I needed anesthesia or if there were a complication I'd be only too happy to have IV and give birth in the delivery room. Peter made it clear that we would be perfectly reasonable if there were complications. The doctor said that if all went well he'd be willing to give it a try. But he was a little dubious about his colleagues' possible reaction to our requests. Anyway, he agreed to talk to them, and told us that he'd try to be there himself. We were impressed, and felt we had chosen the right man.
>
> We took the hospital tour and discussed what we wanted with the head nurse, assuring her that this was our second baby and we were taking classes together. She seemed leery of any change from routine, but she didn't say no. Finally she told us that if it was all right with our doctor, there wouldn't be much problem — even though, as she said a little nervously, "You realize that this hasn't been done before!"
>
> When labor began, we explained that we had our doctor's permission to avoid routine IV; the nurse grumbled a little but didn't push the issue. Fortunately, our own doctor was on: when he arrived he arranged that I would give birth in the labor room. I needed no medication. Peter coached and the doctor was super! I didn't use stirrups . . . the staff couldn't have been nicer and one nurse told us that she wished more couples were

as prepared as we were. We both feel that our birth turned out so well because of all the advance preparation and talking to members of the obstetrical staff.

Like Evelyn and Peter, you can have a say in the way your child is born by working within the existing obstetrical situation — even a relatively conservative one. In the previous chapters we've gone over many of the guidelines for getting the birth of your choice, but I feel they're worth repeating. In this chapter I'll outline 13 basic UPC rules to help you get what you want. All of these have been used effectively by couples in my classes.

Before the birth:
1. Read and investigate.
2. Choose your doctor and hospital carefully.
3. Choose the best possible childbirth preparation course.
4. Go over the details of your birth with the doctor.
5. Choose your pediatrician.

During labor and hospital stay:
6. Use admission forms to give yourself loopholes.
7. Explain to the staff what you're doing.

If things go wrong:
8. Act at the time.
9. Assume that people basically want to help.
10. Be assertive — it's your baby.
11. See the person at the top.
12. If you don't get what you want, write a letter of complaint.

If things go well:
13. Thank the staff.

1. Read and investigate.

Reading a variety of books on childbirth, infant care and parenting will give you a good solid basis for decision making. Particularly outstanding are: *Thank You, Dr. Lamaze,* by Marjorie Karmel, a Dolphin Book by Doubleday, which will give you background on the Lamaze Method; *The Adventure of Birth,* by Elisabeth Bing, Ace Books, a collection of parents' reports of their birth experiences using the Lamaze Method; *Birth Without Violence,* by Frederick Leboyer, Alfred Knopf, discussed earlier in this book; *Birth* by Catherine Milinaire, Harmony Books, Crown Publishers, which outlines various choices in birth "methods", includes parents' accounts and all sorts of bits and pieces on pregnancy and child care with some beautiful photographs; and *Nursing Your Baby,* by Karen Pryor, Pocket Books. (For more recommended reading, check the bibliography at the back of the book.)

At the same time, you can investigate the obstetrical situation in your community. Ask your friends about their own childbirth experiences: if you're lucky, one of them will have experienced PC herself.

If you're new in town, and are really starting from scratch, your best bet in the search for doctor, hospital and classes is to look in the telephone book and see if there's a childbirth education group in the area. Most major centres and many smaller ones have such a group — possibly an associate group of the International Childbirth Education Association (ICEA). If you know some time in advance that you'll be having your baby in another town I'd suggest you write to ICEA at P.O. Box 20852, Milwaukee, Wisconsin, 53220 and request a list of CEA groups and individual members in your area. Members can be a good resource if there is no group — and can also serve as an interested nucleus if you decide to start your own group. The ICEA booklet on *Planning Comprehensive Maternal and Newborn Services for the Childbearing Year* will help in your dialogue with health professionals.

CEA groups are sometimes listed under "Parent

Education'' in the yellow pages. Also, check to see if there's a local chapter of La Leche League International (the breast-feeding information organization). They may be able to provide names of doctors who support Prepared Childbirth — as well as the names of any hospitals with flexible family-centered programs. (Generally, the two go together.) And if none of these approaches give you any leads, try phoning the librarian at your local newspaper as a last resort. Say you are doing research on childbirth in your community and ask to see relevant clippings files. You may be able to turn up a story about PC which will give you the names of a childbirth educator or a doctor who is flexible enough to try this method.

2. Choose your doctor and hospital carefully.

The Doctor. Once you have a few names, proceed using the steps listed in Chapter 6 (The Right to a Supportive Doctor). Make an appointment as soon as possible, because early prenatal care is a must. If you're unable to decide on a doctor or if your appointment is not for some time, routine check-ups, blood tests and urinalysis can be arranged through the outpatients' obstetrical clinic at most large hospitals.

You've used the guidelines and feel fairly satisfied with your doctor — or you have gone "doctor shopping" and have finally found a doctor you feel will allow you choices. Remember that if you have decided to change doctors, do it as soon as possible. Call the doctor you are changing from, explaining your reasons; this action will go a long way towards helping to change that doctor for future couples. Ask that your records be transferred.

What if you're unable to find a doctor who will allow you reasonable choices or who seems noncommittal about things important to you? Suppose you want to be together during the birth: that's the most important thing, you've both agreed. If you can pin him or her down to a definite answer on this point, you're heading the right way. If the doctor still avoids a direct answer, keep talking. Explain that his vagueness is making you anxious — that you'd like to know exactly where you stand. If you're given a, "Most fathers attend the birth as long as everything goes well" reply, try to have the doctor define the conditions under which he would *not* allow you to be together. His reasons may make sense but insist on straight answers on this issue.

If you're still anxious, ask if you could have written permission to be together — particularly helpful if there's a colleague on duty at the time of your birth. (Some doctors will give you a letter; others loathe the very mention of "written".) If you've explained yourselves and given the doctor every chance to discuss the issues with you and you still feel uneasy — *change!* But if this doctor seems the most flexible available, try to discuss your feelings at each visit and keep on trying. As long as the doctor seems to support the father's presence, you'll probably get what you want.

If you're a single mother who will be accompanied by another woman throughout labor, discuss this with the doctor and make sure that you and your friend will be together — often a written consent will clear the way for you in labor. It is *vitally important* that you and your coach be together at every phase of labor and that staff and doctor clearly understand that she will be present.

The Hospital. You've chosen your doctor. Now it's time to check out the hospital. Use the guidelines in Chapter 10, and arrange your tour as soon as possible. If you're reasonably sure that your hospital stay will be based on your needs, then you now have both your doctor and hospital.

If your hospital appears extremely rigid and you feel that your needs will not be met in several areas which you feel are important, speak to the obstetrical supervisor. I have found that this person is usually extremely anxious to help and a sensible discussion with her of what you are looking for and why will probably go a long way in your favour. You may find, as Evelyn and Peter did, that your request has simply never been made before.

If you are told that your requests are impossible (complete

rooming-in, say) and they are very important to you, try discussing the situation with your doctor. If that doesn't seem to help, you can try calling another hospital — and again ask for the obstetrical supervisor. It's a lot of effort, but worth it if you find a sympathetic hospital. Of course, you'll probably need a new doctor if you switch hospitals, so ask for names of doctors affiliated with the hospital, check with your original contact (CEA group, La Leche, etc.) and see if they can recommend one of the names on the list. Or ask the obstetrical supervisor for a doctor who will fit in with your needs. These actions are all highly unorthodox — but many couples have used them effectively. Remember that organizing things in advance will spare you all sorts of problems later. One woman jokingly remarked at a class one night, "It's a good thing pregnancy is so long — I needed all that time to find a doctor and hospital we were comfortable with!"

If you can't find your ideal hospital but have come up with one which meets several of your needs and seems fairly flexible, you'll probably decide to stick with it and concentrate on getting as much as you can during your hospital stay — or at worst, arranging home help and a short stay.

3. Choose the best possible childbirth preparation course.

You've now chosen a doctor and a hospital that you're fairly confident you can work with. Your next step is to enrol in your preparation course. Use the guidelines given in Chapter 7. Ideally the doctor, hospital and course are all geared to similar goals and should all be familiar with each other.

Situation hopeless?

You're new to town and there isn't a CEA and you can't find a PC course or a doctor or hospital who'll give you any flexibility in childbirth. The situation isn't quite so hopeless as it seems. If you don't have much time to act — your baby is due soon — your best plan of action is to find one medical

professional who supports Prepared Childbirth, and start
from there. Ask around: a call to a women's group, the nursing school at a college or university nearby, may unearth the
name of a suitable doctor. Talking with other women — in
your neighborhood, at work, almost any place — may prove
helpful. Once you've found the doctor, getting together with
a group of other couples interested in Prepared Childbirth
may start things rolling at a pace which will surprise you.

An advertisement in a local newspaper, or posters an-
nouncing a meeting for anyone interested in Prepared Childbirth or the Lamaze Method or anything else you want to call
it has been shown to get results. Put up posters in community
halls, schools, day care centres, shopping centres and I
guarantee you'll have at least one or two calls within a day or
so.

Nancy and Eric P., members of the Montreal CEA decided
to take matters into their own hands in a "hopeless" situation. Nancy wrote to the newsleter of MCEA:

> *We enjoyed the CEA so much in Montreal that we
> hoped to continue our efforts, learning and enthusiasm
> upon our move to (a certain city) two years ago. Alas,
> not only was there no such vibrant and vital
> organization, but nowhere could we find a Lamaze
> teacher to instruct me in the breathing and relaxation I
> needed for the birth of my second child. Finally I found
> a fellow disenchanted soul, expecting her baby like me,
> and looking for a refresher course in Lamaze, after
> having had excellent instruction in another city two
> years earlier. We teamed up, she taught me everything
> she knew and the outcome was a great success.*

> *However, two years later, the situation remains the
> same here. A so-called "Childbirth Education" group
> exists but they stress that they don't like to limit them-
> selves to one method or teach any one theory. And
> because they do not "believe in" anything in particular,
> these negative attitudes quickly transferred to the*

student couples in the classes they give.

Compare this with the total psychological and physical involvement of Lamaze and the extremely positive reactions and reinforcement the method provides for both man and woman! Where else but at a Lamaze birth could a potentially painful experience become a joyful challenge, even fun half-the-time, and give you the satisfaction that you've done it together?

We need a Lamaze organization here, and people qualified to give the training . . . I am interested in hearing from anyone who has any thoughts on this matter . . .

The response to Nancy's letter was excellent. Several MCEA couples from my classes were moving to the same city; they joined with Nancy to form a group and found one doctor and a nurse who were interested in Lamaze. Nancy wrote to ASPO (American Society of Psychoprophylaxis in Obstetrics) and embarked on its training course. Recently, she became a qualified Lamaze instructor and the one doctor has spread his enthusiasm around the hospital where he works. Other nurses and members of the medical profession have become interested and now a wave of enthusiasm for the method is spreading across the city.

If you discover, as Nancy and Eric did, that in order to get PC classes going you have to — somehow — organize them yourself, write to ICEA for help. They will be able to give you all sorts of invaluable information on setting up a group.

What if it's "too late"?

Or suppose that your baby is due in a few weeks and you can't find a preparation course. I'd suggest you talk with your doctor. Tell him that you'd like to use PC, and ask him about the situation at the hospital where he works. You may still be able to get what you want. If it appears that the doctor will simply not listen, you still have time to locate a more supportive doctor via the sources I've mentioned above — a last resort if you're close to due date! If it's too late to enrol in a course, I'd suggest you get hold of the excellent paperback *Six Practical Lessions For An Easier Childbirth* by Elisabeth Bing — a practical manual in the Lamaze method for you and your partner. I've sent this book to couples in remote areas and they've reported great success!

4.   Go over details of the birth with your doctor.

Suppose you now have a doctor, hospital and childbirth preparation course more or less to your liking. You have visited your hospital together; your reading plus the knowledge acquired in classes is giving you an excellent basis for questions and choices. As birth approaches, I'd recommend that mother and father attend one or two visits to the doctor together, and go over the details of the birth. Even if you've already discussed this with your doctor earlier, it helps to make details clear in the last few weeks.

But what if you're a little uneasy about your doctor's colleagues? You've asked about them and your doctor has assured you that they all share his/her obstetrical policies — they're couple-oriented, flexible and open to variations. Perhaps you've decided that you'd prefer not to use stirrups and that you would like episiotomy to be assessed on a need basis rather than performed routinely. Your doctor says there'll be no problem with him, but seems just a little non-committal about Colleagues A and B. You might admit you're worried. Ask if you could rotate with the other doctors in the group to meet briefly with each. Some couples find it reassuring to have a note from the doctor to the effect that permission has been given to avoid stirrups etc. The paper may not be necessary but you know it's there in case you need it.

Some doctors refuse to sign anything. If that's the case, you need to talk things over until you know exactly where you stand. As we've discussed in Chapter 6, you might decide to compromise on some details as long as you have the most important elements of PC. It's crucial that you clear everything in advance! Find out what you can and cannot have before labor. Don't wait until you're hiccupping and fiercely concentrating on the all absorbing beat of "Yankee Doodle" in the hour before birth, to ask about the way the birth is to be managed — you won't feel like discussing things then at all! The last thing either of you will feel like at this point is explaining your philosophy on couple-oriented childbirth.

5. Choose Your Pediatrician.

If you have not chosen a pediatrician for your baby by the time of birth, the newborn checkup will be done routinely by the hospital's resident pediatrician. However, if you have chosen one in advance, he or she can help you enormously by leaving specific instructions on your baby's chart. For example, specifying, "No supplements" or "baby rooming-in" can clear the way at a hospital where these procedures are rare. If you are delivering your baby at a hospital with fairly rigid policies, a pediatrician who supports family-centred maternity care can work wonders.

One of my clients, Angela, planned to deliver her baby at a hospital where there is a routine 24-hour observation period, and where all babies are supplemented with formula in the nursery. She was planning to breastfeed and wanted to nurse immediately after birth, and have rooming-in with no supplements. She phoned her pediatrician for a prenatal appointment; the nurse told her such appointments weren't necessary but arranged one anyway. Later, Angela told me:

> *The pediatrician wasn't too enthusiastic about what I wanted, but when I explained* why, *she said she saw no reason for my not having complete rooming-in with no supplements. I asked if she would leave instructions on the chart. She said she'd never been asked to do this before, but sure, why not? I had the baby in my room, no supplements were given, and there was no hassle because the order came from the pediatrician.*

Many of the guidelines to choosing your obstetrician apply here — but here are some additional guidelines:

Does he or she see couples prenatally? Some do, often with a group of other couples. Such visits are a helpful way of finding out his or her ideas — for example, on infant feeding.

Does he or she encourage breastfeeding? "Do many of your clients breastfeed?" will give you an answer which tells you a lot about his/her approach to the subject. If you're planning to breastfeed, it's essential to have a pediatrician who is supportive. Too many pediatricians are geared to a majority of bottle-fed babies, and will suggest supplementary bottles or a complete use of the bottle if you encounter the slightest problem in nursing. Even if the pediatrician does not provide a prenatal visit, you may be able to arrange one or at least have your questions answered before the baby is born.

Is he or she affiliated with the hospital where you're giving birth? This is helpful, especially in establishing good breastfeeding routines, as I pointed out earlier. But if you happen to have the rare luxury of a true family doctor who, unfortunately, isn't connected with your hospital, it's usually worthwhile to stick with him or her — and let the resident pediatrician do the newborn checkup.

Does this pediatrician have evening office hours? Some do, these days — and this is a real boon to nine-to-five working parents.

Consider location, too. If you happen to live in Canada or the northern U.S., it's useful to choose a pediatrician whose office is easily accessible in bad weather. (Few things are more harrowing than a one-hour ride in a snowstorm with a sick child!)

If you don't have names of pediatricians recommended by friends, you can get a few names from your obstetrician. Or call in at the children's hospital in your area if there is one; an information officer should be able to give you a list of pediatricians affiliated there.

6. Use admission forms to give yourself loopholes.

Finally you're in labor. You've spent four hours at home and you've been using breathing techniques for the last hour or so. You've taken a leisurely trip to the hospital: you're excited, nervous, but outwardly calm. You and your partner are working together as you've learned. But now you're faced with the irritating details of admission. You've asked to pre-register but there's still a form left which you have been told can only be filled out at the time of actual arrival.

Instead of looking at this form (or forms) as one more irritation, view it as an escape hatch. You can use it to give yourself leeway in refusing what you consider unnecessary routines. Usually you are required to sign a "consent form", even if you're almost ready to give birth! In many cases, the father is asked to complete this for his partner on admission. Nicette and Tibor used the admission form to ensure that routines were subject to their "informed consent". Nicette explains:

> *We had spent considerable time choosing a doctor, hospital and classes, and we felt that we knew enough to make decisions about the birth. When we arrived at the hospital I had to sign a three-clause form. My husband was asked to sign for me while I was being prepped but he refused to sign until I had seen the form. An intern brought me the form and told me that it was "just routine" but why bother having signatures if you don't even read it?*
>
> *The first part of the form gave permission for routine treatment and medical procedures. The second gave permission for surgery — under that had been penned in "delivery and episiotomy" and the third, for anesthesia. Because one of the doctors in the group likes to give gas during the actual birth, and had given it to a friend a while ago, without her permission, I was taking no chances. I signed all three clauses but under the*

> *third, added, "medication, analgesia and anesthesia to*
> *be given only on request and with adequate explanation*
> *of need."*
>
> *I think the staff were irritated, but I was glad that I*
> *had done that because Doctor Gas was on duty, and I*
> *didn't have any medication.*

Valerie and Serge Poulard didn't see the need for routine fetal monitoring or an IV, because Valerie was not a high-risk pregnancy. When Valerie signed the form, she added, "all procedures to be carried out only with my complete understanding of the need for such." The Poulards were at a hospital where IV's and monitors are used almost routinely, and Valerie bypassed them because of this clause: instead, the fetal heart rate was monitored by a nurse.

The "subject to my complete understanding of procedures involved" clause is useful if you want to avoid any of the hospital "routines". But be careful to make your decisions after careful thought, to avoid "faddiness" and be aware that in sidestepping routine you take on yourselves responsibility for anything which goes wrong. (I have never heard of a case where bypassing a routine led to anything undesirable.) In the event of a complication, medical staff should explain procedures so that you give your "informed consent" with full understanding of the need.

"In my case the clause was a safeguard because as it turned out I did not have to resort to it", says Valerie. "The nurses were surprised when I told them that I had the doctor's permission to bypass routines. They respected our decisions and were supportive — except for one nurse who really wanted to shave me, something I had requested not be done. When it's all boiled down, nobody can force you into these procedures."

Serge P. adds:

> *Parents who want to do as we did must be aware that*
> *they're shouldering responsibility if anything goes*

wrong. Don't do anything lightly, do it only if it's important to you and you've researched the pros and cons. Also start your research early in pregnancy. If you know in advance that you'll be going against routines you must start talking as early as possible to the people who'll be there.

7. Explain to the staff what you're doing.

You've cleared with your doctor any routines which you've chosen to avoid but it's not your doctor who's on duty. Right from the start you'll avoid possible misunderstandings if you explain basically what you're doing to the nurse, intern and resident as soon as you arrive. Perhaps you've been given your doctor's OK to stay together for admission procedures. An explanation to the nurse is absolutely necessary! Something along the lines of "We'd really like to stay together for everything and we've discussed it with our doctor. We have his/her permission and we realize it's not routine but it's very important to us", will usually clear the way.

A note to the father: Perhaps you've decided that it's not terribly important to remain with your partner during the "prep". Labor may be moving slowly, but you have your doctor's permission to remain for everything. If more than 30 minutes have gone by, put on the gown hanging in the fathers' room and go into the labor area! If staff are busy, this action may shorten your wait outside. If you are told that you can't come in, explain that you have permission. You might use the approach, "I know it's not routine and we realize you might be embarrassed but if you really don't mind we'd like to be together."

In the case of a potentially non-supportive staff member, it's best to explain as early as possible in the labor what you're doing and ask for his or her support: a brief explanation on arrival to the nurse, intern and resident may help you avoid a misunderstanding later. You might say, "We're using the Lamaze method. When I have a contraction it helps if I concentrate on my breathing — so I'd really appreciate it if you could wait until it's over to ask questions." Or "I've prepared with my wife and I'll be able to help with her breathing. We'd really like to be allowed to work together during each contraction." Or "I'm not decided one way or the other about anesthetic, but please don't mention it unless I really feel I need something." This last comment will save you many well-meant offers of something to "help you relax" or "take the edge off things"; it also clarifies the fact that you are not attempting to be a *martyr,* suffering to achieve a goal of no medication — (an idea firmly embedded in the minds of many staff members).

The best approach, which I have rarely found to fail, is "We're confident that you are here to help us and we'll cooperate if you will" — much more positive than communicating a feeling of "us versus you". Remember, you are dealing with people who basically do want to help! Even a supportive member of staff can have a bad day; treating him/her pleasantly is only going to improve things for all of you.

Having established that most medical personnel feel they have your best interests at heart, I now must add that until every member of the staff is familiar with the prepared couple, there is always a chance of apathy, non-support or misunderstanding. And no matter how well you plan in advance, occasionally there's a problem at the last minute — possibly one staff member whose attitude threatens to undermine all your efforts. If you don't know how to respond, chances are much of your hard work is in vain. Because the woman in labor is caught up in body rhythms and work, she is usually unable to handle such unexpected problems — so the coach must be prepared to deal with the offending staff member. Rules 8 to 11 will help deal with last minute hassles.

8.   Act at the time.

Even at a hospital where you're fairly sure you'll have the sort of birth you'd like, you may be dismayed to run into one member of staff who does not reflect what you've been told is the general attitude of the hospital. After the birth of their baby, David C. told a class of their experience:

> *All the other staff members had respected what we were doing, but this one nurse came in and told Karen she was doing her breathing "all wrong" and she would help her baby more if she had an epidural. We had been working together for about three hours and Karen had felt very much on top of things. We'd discussed in class that staff members might become upset if they saw a woman hyperventilating, but Karen was not doing that at all — she was not in pain, either. When the nurse said that I could almost see Karen thinking, "What's the use?"*

> *Hospitals are intimidating, but it was either say something or watch Karen lose control. I stepped outside and explained to the nurse that we had spend considerable time preparing with this method and that it was helping Karen. I told her I knew that sometimes women hyperventilated, but Karen was not likely to run into this problem. I added that she probably hadn't intended to upset Karen, but she had — and would she please not make any more comments?*

> *She was obviously taken aback, and said, "Well — you do what you've learned" and after that she left us alone. After the birth I thanked her.*

It's vital that you act at the time! Remember that although, as David said, hospitals can be pretty intimidating, you probably only have a child a few times in a lifetime, maybe only once. To allow some small incident to spoil your efforts can be terribly upsetting — and it's almost always preventable.

If the woman is unable to work up the nerve to complain, the father should be able to. He's in a better position in several ways. He's more mobile — can walk to the desk. He's also not so totally absorbed in the physical and emotional stress of birth, so he's slightly less vulnerable.

What do you do if polite attempts don't work? Richard told me about the situation he and Betty encountered:

> *There was an intern who seemed determined to sabotage our efforts. He made condescending remarks while we were working together and everything he said was a put-down, even though we'd politely explained what we were doing . . . He continued harping until Betty was almost in tears. I told him that he had made his point perfectly clear and could he please leave? He did. It left a bad taste but at least Betty and I were left alone to work in peace.*

9.   Assume people basically want to help.

Fortunately, however, staff members who are directly antagonistic are rare. Most nurses, medical trainees and doctors do not want to upset you, and most are anxious to make things easier. You have a right to expect courteous treatment from all staff, as they have a right to expect the same from you. For example, if a staff member comes in and asks you to position for an internal, without so much as an introduction, you are quite justified in saying, "I don't think we know who you are." It's sometimes helpful for you, the father, to approach it along the lines of, "I'm John Doe, I don't think we've met. . ." If examinations are unnecessarily uncomfortable, say so! "I'm finding this uncomfortable, could you please be more gentle?" should do the trick.

Often a straightforward, "I know you're trying to help and we appreciate that, but. . ." may work wonders. Although hospitals can be intimidating, try to look at a hassle in perspective. As long as you're reasonably polite, nothing terrible is going to happen if you're firm. You have everything to gain, nothing to lose. You don't have to be rude, just insistent. You're dealing with normal, usually pleasant people. There are no ogres in case rooms (usually!) but sometimes there are tired, overworked people who may at the time of your labor have problems which make them less sensitive to your needs.

There's a chance you may arrive at the hospital in rush hour. Even a hospital which normally is flexible and supportive of Prepared Childbirth tends to become less than ideal during a very busy period. It helps in this case to let the staff know you appreciate the fact that they're rushed. "It must be terribly hard being so busy", Victor B. told the case room nurse assigned to his wife, "We really appreciate the help you're giving us. If there's anything I can do to help let me know . . ." Later he told me:

> *The nurse couldn't have been nicer after that. After the baby was born, I knew they were rushed and it seemed that they were going to whisk the baby away without a cuddle. I told the nurse, "I know how busy you are, but we've been looking forward to holding our baby for months," and she gave her to us. Afterwards, another couple — who also had their baby during rush period — complaind to me that they hadn't even been given the baby to hold. But you've got to do more than just sit there and expect everything you want without any effort, particularly when you see that everybody is frantically busy.*

10.   Be assertive — it's your baby.

The E's wanted to avoid the use of stirrups at delivery, also episiotomy if at all possible. Jan had had no medication and was fully in control. Her doctor's colleague was on duty and she saw him briefly for an internal just before delivery:

> *I was wheeled into the delivery room and the nurses automatically started to adjust the stirrups. I'd meant to discuss this with the colleague but you're under far too much stress then. Fortunately Ed had spoken to the doctor just as they were walking to the delivery room and Dr. B. said to the nurses, "It's OK — they've cleared it*

with me" and all went well. If Ed hadn't mentioned it I
think I would have just gone along with the stirrups
because you can't argue and don't feel like explaining
just as you're about to give birth.

Have your partner speak to the doctor as soon as he arrives
and explain that you're prepared; that you have your own
doctor's consent and you'll co-operate as much as he wants
you to if he feels it's medically necessary. As I've noted
earlier, if you want to breastfeed immediately after delivery;
avoid or minimize observation period; have flexible feeding
schedules or complete "rooming-in", you should discuss
these desires with the doctor and hospital staff in advance. If
possible, have your pediatrician write these requests on your
chart. But if, during or after childbirth, it seems that staff are
ignoring your previously discussed wishes, *speak up* — or ask
the baby's father to do it if he is feeling more assertive than
you are. What have you got to lose? All they can say is NO.

Don't take No for an answer.
Note to the father: You've made it through to delivery,
you're already changed into father's gear for delivery. Your
partner's doctor is not on duty. Colleague A. arrives and
gives you a hasty, "Sorry, but I'm afraid you'll have to wait
outside."
You're terribly upset; so far the labor has seemed normal.
Don't leave! Say something like, "I'm sorry, Doctor, but
there's a misunderstanding — we have our doctor's permission to be together and he told us that you would be as
supportive as he is. I'm fully prepared and won't get in the
way."
If he refuses, ask if there is a complication, or if this is his
usual policy. His action probably is a whim of the moment or
your doctor would have warned you. It may be simply that
the birth is moving along quickly and he hasn't really given it
a thought. I've spoken to many couples to whom this has occurred, usually when the area is busy. All but one of the men

insisted that they go in — nobody threw them out and there were no apparent hard feelings. George Y. did not push the issue, and two years later he's still bitter. "I wish I'd just gone in", he told me when he and his wife began preparing for their second child.

Fortunately, such cases are becoming rare, but it can happen. If you've cleared everything in advance there is usually no problem, but should one arise be firm. Refusing to take no for an answer won't make you popular with the staff — but it can get a father into the delivery room, or a baby out of a lengthy observation period in the nursery and into the arms of her mother. In getting your own way, however, use creative, tactful stubbornness rather than downright aggressiveness. Strive to present an image of a cool, calm, responsible and confident parent. (One good reason why the father is usually the best person to deal with hospital hassles: a woman in labor is in no condition to play diplomat!)

11. See the person at the top.

If the previous rules seem to have no effect, you have nothing to lose by going straight to the top. If you've chosen your hospital with an eye to flexibility, the head nurse or obstetrical supervisor will usually be eager to promote a more client-oriented and family-centered approach. For example, Martin and Liz I. had been assured by their doctor that they could be together during every procedure. But when they arrived at the labor room, the nurse asked Martin to go to the fathers' room until Liz — who was already having strong contractions — was "ready". Martin explained that they had their doctor's permission to be together, but the nurse was adamant. So Martin asked to see the supervisor and told the nurse he would wait outside until she arrived:

> *I was really surprised when the supervisor appeared. She was extremely pleasant — and told me that because we had our doctor's permission, she would speak to the nurse. A few minutes later, the nurse came out and*

fetched me, and I remained with Liz until the baby was born — even though I could see the nurse thought I was some sort of crank!

Mrs. H. chose her hospital because it was proud of its family-centered maternity care. She had been told she could nurse her baby immediately after birth and have him four hours later in her room for complete rooming-in if both mother and baby were healthy. She got what she wanted — but only after going to the top.

I felt fine, nursed my baby on the delivery table and four hours later asked for him. The nurse told me that I needed my rest and that there was no rush, I'd have my baby "soon enough" and why didn't I just get my rest?

I didn't feel sleepy. I wanted my baby. Another two hours went by. Finally out of desperation I rang and asked for the head nurse. She came and was very understanding and said there was no reason why I couldn't have my baby. Within fifteen minutes I had him.

12.   If you don't get what you want, write a letter of complaint.

By far, your best approach is to speak to the people concerned at the time, when things go wrong. But even if you are unable to bring yourself to complain at the time, because you're afraid of souring the staff to you, a letter may help change things for future couples — or future pregnancies. Louise Rothmar wrote such a letter:

On (date) I delivered a lovely baby girl at (hospital).

I want to say that the caseroom staff were exceptionally wonderful people. The experience for my husband and me will remain one of joy and happiness with wonderful people helping . . .

I am a firm believer in breastfeeding and was completely equipped with all the knowledge necessary to

become a successful nursing mother, but I found the nurses' information and advice on this to be contrary to everything I had learned from other successfully nursing mothers and several excellent books on breastfeeding
. . .

I found it difficult in the first two days to find a nurse who would agree to let me have my baby on a demand feeding schedule. I was told, "You don't have much to offer your baby until your milk comes in. Glucose and water are better for her now." The maternity staff were overloaded but there is no valid reason why the new mother should suffer. Couldn't you help us nursing mothers with more encouragement? It would be appreciated so much and help make breastfeeding a success. Thank you for taking time out of a busy work day.

This letter had an immediate effect. The obstetrical supervisor called me about the letter, as a copy had been sent to me, and it was I who suggested a letter might help. We arranged to visit Louise and another woman with similar complaints, and the head nurse went too. We discussed the content of the letter — the problems which a busy staff may face, and some of the ways which might be used to encourage breastfeeding mothers. The results were dramatic and almost instantaneous. Reports from women delivering at this hospital have been unanimously enthusiastic about the care and support of the nurses for breastfeeding.

If you have a complaint about childbirth or post-natal care, such a letter is invaluable. If you decide to write, do so as soon as possible after the event. Direct it to the nursing supervisor, or — if the complaint deals with a doctor, intern or resident — to the obstetrical chief. A short letter stating what you liked, what you found unhelpful or upsetting, following details as date, room number and names of persons involved is usually most effective.

13. Thank the staff

Hospital staffs enjoy hearing from you not only when you have constructive criticism, but also when you feel the care has been exceptionally good. Staffs are subjected to much criticism. If you've had a good experience, they would love to hear from you. Janice M. was delighted by her hospital experience and wrote the following letter, some months after Louise had delivered at the same hospital:

> *I have nothing but praise for the professionalism of your staff and the great flexibility of your system. I think I tested both to the fullest. I wanted childbirth without medication using the Lamaze techniques — followed by complete rooming-in so that I could breast-feed on demand.*
>
> *I was hostile when I went in. I expected to be dealing with staff who did not sympathize with these things. Your staff succeeded in "taming" me with their great professionalism, competence, perception and teamwork.*

These paragraphs were followed by a list of the individual people who had made her experience so memorable. Positive letters reinforce helpful behaviour on the part of the staff — and can go a long way towards implementing progressive hospital policies. Although obstetrical systems do not change overnight I've been amazed at how quickly the hospital staffs have responded to couples' requests and follow-up letters. The obstetrical system in the community where you live might at this time be less than adequate, but the only way to create an ideal similar to those I'll discuss in the next chapter is to make an effort yourself. If a significant number of people request change, the system will respond. Not only will your action get you the childbirth of your choice, but you'll make it easier for the women and men who come after you.

12

It's everybody's baby

Gourmet OB Recipe: Joyous Childbirth A La Lamaze

To an attractive, home-like labor-delivery room add:

1. One enthusiastic couple properly prepared in the Lamaze method by an ASPO certified instructor.

2. One Lamaze "bag of tricks" with lollipop, chapstick, face cloth, corn starch, playing cards, notebook, pencil, camera, sandwich, thermos and list of 'phone numbers.

3. One comfortable, versatile labor-delivery bed.

4. One enthusiastic OB nurse trained in the Lamaze method (monitrice) to run the room and provide constant, uninterrupted support (verbal analgesia) throughout labor and delivery.

5. One enthusiastic obstetrician.

6. One paracervical-block tray to reduce intensity of sensation if necesary.

Add appropriate medical equipment. Add a spot of spunk, a smidgen of spirit, a cup of cussedness and a large dollup of determination.

Decorate with colorful wallpaper, drapes, pictures, mobiles, AM-FM radio, delivery mirror, telephone, Polaroid camera and champagne glasses.

Garnish with grins, lace with love.

Place near a D.R. and O.R. in event of complication.

Baking time 30 mins. to 12 hours. Satisfaction guaranteed!

> *— From a pamphlet issued to prospective*
> *parents by*
> *Manchester Memorial Hospital, Connecticut.*

In our search for obstetrical ideals, David and I visited Manchester Memorial Hospital in Manchester, Connecticut in November, 1975. After viewing the French and Dutch labor-delivery rooms, we were delighted to learn that a Manchester obstetrician, Dr. Philip Sumner, had introduced a similar concept to the United States. Dr. Sumner had visited France in 1969 and toured the Chateau Belvedere with Dr. Pierre Vellay. The combination labor-delivery room appealed to him and some time later he was responsible for bringing a French labor-delivery bed to Manchester.

Our guide was Billie Carlston, R.N., a key force in preparing couples in the Lamaze method and implementing the program at the hospital. "Originally fathers were not permitted at delivery here," she told us. "Then Lamaze-trained couples asked whether they could remain in the labor room to be together. There wasn't a suitable labor room so we converted a storage room. The idea caught on quickly and soon we had the labor-delivery bed."

She showed us the three labor-delivery rooms — bright and friendly, with coloured walls, curtains, pictures and mobiles. Each couple is assigned a nurse on admission, and European-style, she stays with them right through the birth. "There are thirteen registered nurses who act as monitrices, and we're each on call for a twenty-four hour stretch on a rotation basis,'' Billie Carlston told us.

The father remains for the entire labor and birth and is regarded as an integral member of the team. As birth approaches, modified French "ball and socket" stirrups are attached to the sides of the bed so that the woman can choose a comfortable stirrup position. The upper part of the bed can be raised to any comfortable angle, and, as in France, the lower segment of the bed is pushed under the middle segment and regular draping carried out. After birth, the baby is given to its parents at once. Mother, father and baby remain together for about an hour after birth, with the nurse close at hand.

We were shown plastic champagne glasses used to celebrate the birth, and a Polaroid camera which parents can use to snap an instant portrait of their newborn. Each labor room has a large book in which the nurse on duty records details of labor and suitable comments about the couples' feelings at birth. We were delighted to read enthusiastic comments such as "Fantastic birth with relaxed couple" . . . "Couple elated" . . . "A beautiful birth!"

Not all the doctors on staff use the new rooms — in fact, only three use it routinely. But those three are extremely positive about their results. Dr. Sumner believes that perinatal morbidity and mortality is lower in labor-delivery rooms and says the Caesarean rate is half that of the births which proceed along traditional lines.

Because Lamaze-trained women need less medication, only prepared couples may use these labor-delivery rooms. These rooms do not have general anesthesia facilities although they are equipped with fetal heart monitors and standard incubators.

Of the first 800 Lamaze-trained women who used the facilities, 94% gave birth in the room; 4% were transferred to the regular delivery room for vaginal delivery and 2% of the babies were born by Caesarean. Out of the 32 vaginal deliveries transferred, two gave birth spontaneously, but had been moved because of possible need for anaesthesia; 18 were delivered with forceps and there were five breech presentations. The condition of the infants born in the Lamaze room was excellent — an astonishing average of 9.9 out of a possible 10 on the Apgar neonatal assessment scale. (An infant scoring 6 or more is considered healthy.) [1]

The Birth Room

By the late '70s, we had managed to bring many changes to Montreal's birthing community. But there was little provision for home birth, and hospital procedures were unattractive to parents who were searching for home birth. While a group of lay midwives and a handful of doctors were gaining momentum with home birth services, it became apparent that more alternatives were necessary in hospitals.

In May, 1978, as a result of several meetings with parents' groups, Dr. Morrie Gelfand, chief of obstetrics at the Mortimer B. Davis Jewish General Hospital, asked me to set up the Birth Room program. This hospital has a fine reputation for its neonatology unit, high-risk care, and low perinatal mortality rate. However, there was no childbirth education program, and actively managed labor was the norm.

The hospital had plans for new construction in the obstetrical wing. It would be possible to include plans for a living room-bedroom birth room — a matter of knocking out a wall between an existing labor room and an adjoining office.

The first step was setting up a complete childbirth education program. I began such a program, offering sessions in early pregnancy, continuing in mid- and then late pregnancy, and following through into parenting classes after the birth. I also set up sessions to train instructors. Concurrent with the parent classes went classes for staff, until every member of the obstetrical team was familiar with techniques taught in classes and could work with parents. In-service education sessions for staff included slides of European birth, a film of a labor room birth, and films of home birth. We spent many hours talking about staff feelings and attitudes. Support for prepared parents increased.

In June, 1979, my husband David and I spent a glorious morning in a furniture warehouse. We chose a big brass bed (so that parents could rest in labor, and to allow parents and baby to cuddle in bed after the birth); a brown corduroy hide-a-bed, should a support person need to rest in the course of labor; several coffee tables; a braided carpet; and a huge, comfortable rocking chair.

Finally the room was ready. Despite its location in a large general hospital, it provided a distinctly homey atmosphere. But more important than the physical setting is the philosophy which accompanies the birth room: *birth is a normal, healthy event, which with adequate preparation and staff support can occur in a home-like setting without active management.*

The parents who have used the birth room to date have had, I think, everything they hoped for. All parents must be prepared and be screened as "low risk". Friends and family may also attend. The fetal heart rate is taken by the nurse, a vitally important support person. Electronic monitoring has no place in the room unless there is a medical indication picked up in labor. In this case, a monitor can be used for a limited time, and removed. If there is a problem the mother is transferred to a regular labor room. Shaves, enemas, IVs and medication are not used in the birth room.

Mothers are encouraged to move freely and use a comfortable position for birth (sitting, squatting, kneeling). Parents and baby remain in the birth room for an hour after birth to cuddle, nurse, and get to know each other, with full staff backup.

Some mothers have developed complications in labor and have been transferred to an adjacent delivery room. All were prepared for this possibility, and did not find that it marred their birth experience. Because the birth room is part of a comprehensive childbirth program it has benefited all births at the hospital. It is more than some nice furniture and pretty curtains; it is the embodiment of the philosophy of the non-managed birth. Thanks to the hours of discussion and staff training that went into the birth room program, it is recognized as such by all members of the professional staff, regardless of how they feel about intervention in childbirth.

This birth room was the first of its kind in Canada, though McMaster Medical Centre in Hamilton, Ontario has offered parents a similar experience in the austere surrounding of a regular labor room for some years. Putting the birth room program in place was one of the more difficult tasks I have faced in childbirth education — not so much designing the room as inculcating the philosophy behind it. Without that philosophy, the managed birth will dominate, regardless of the setting. It is my hope that more birth room programs will be started across the continent.

Home Birth:
The Uneasy Alternative

With the improvements we've seen recently, maternal mortality is now practically zero in this state (California) and newborn infant mortality has been reduced from about 20 per 1,000 live births to 14 per thousand in the past five or six years. That's a very dramatic improvement and it's not going to be maintained if we go in the direction of more home delivery.

> — *Dr. Thomas Elmendorf,*
> *past president,*
> *California Medical Association.*[2]

In recent years, probably the most controversial trend in obstetrics has been the return to home birth for a growing number of couples, disenchanted with the managed hospital birth. Quoted in an article in the *Toronto Globe and Mail,* two British Columbia doctors condemn this trend:

> *If the whole community is geared to home deliveries with . . . trained midwives, sterile portable bundles, ready access to pre-arranged hospital back-up facilities, flying squads and ambulances . . . that is one thing.*
> *But if these are not organized and available, home deliveries are unacceptable.[3]*

"Back-up" is the crucial word. In most of North America, we simply don't have it. In my opinion, the ideal obstetrical system combines safety with flexibility and choice. I am not familiar with the Scottish system described by Alice C., but judging from her report, it would seem to approach the ideal. So does the system in Holland, which I outlined in Chapter 1. A woman in the Netherlands may choose between birth at home, if the pregnancy is normal — with superb prenatal care and a trained midwife at the birth — or a flexible hospital birth with constant support, and little or no interference with normal labor. If she chooses hospital birth, she may return home after 24 hours with follow-up midwife visits, or remain in hospital for a full seven days.

All women classified as "high-risk" give birth in hospital. All women see an obstetrician at least once during the pregnancy, but may visit a midwife or general practitioner for regular care. High-risk pregnancies are carefully screened. More than 85% of all Dutch women attend childbirth preparation classes, and the importance of good nutrition is stressed from the beginning of pregnancy. About 60% of Dutch women give birth at home: Holland's low mortality rate among newborn infants attests to the safety of a well organized home birth system for normal birth.

Britain and some other European countries also provide home birth as a safe alternative with "flying squads" — mobile units fitted with emergency equipment which can be on hand at a moment's notice. In these countries, most normal home births are attended by a trained nurse-midwife, and her role is a vital one.

In North America, the home birth movement is rapidly

gaining strength. Organizations which prepare women for safe home birth and provide trained attendants and medical back-up are mushrooming. Early studies suggest the trend is a healthy one — though without support services its future is limited.

In California, 287 home births, attended by lay midwives with limited medical backup, were studied by a group of four members of a health research team from Stanford University and the University of California. The births occurred between 1971 and 1973 under direction of the Santa Cruz Birth Center. All women received good prenatal care, nutrition was uniformly good and each birth was attended by two midwives. All women attended childbirth preparation classes, and breastfed their children.

231 births were completely normal, and the rate of complications was lower than for the population as a whole. Complications occurred in 56 women and 45 of these required medical intervention in hospital for completion of delivery. There was one stillborn baby, but no deaths of babies born live. The infection rate following childbirth was 1.8%, comparable to infection rates in hospital births.[4]

The results of the study show that neonatal mortality and morbidity were lower in an unanesthetized natural childbirth population than in the population as a whole. The team attributed the success of home birth in this study to the preparedness of the women, lack of analgesics and anesthetics, the avoidance of the supine birth position (semisitting, hands-and-knees position and side-lying were popular positions) and to the absence of obstetrical interference and unnecessary routines.

Organizations to prepare couples for safe home birth have developed in the last few years in North America. Among them is a Washington D.C. group called H.O.M.E. (Home Oriented Maternity Experience), which lists as prerequisites for a safe and healthy home birth:

1. intention to nurse the baby.

2. excellent prenatal care.
3. above average nutrition.
4. no previous high risk pregnancies, labors or deliveries.
(A seemingly wise fifth precaution is taken in many European countries — Britain among them, as Alice C. pointed out. Mothers are encouraged to birth the first baby in hospital. If all goes well, they may consider home birth for successive children.)
H.O.M.E. urges couples to attend childbirth preparation classes with a teacher familiar with and in favour of home delivery. It stresses that home birth requires a "high degree of participation, responsibility and personal commitment from the couple to ensure that their needs and the needs of the child are met."

Pediatrician Russell J. Bunai agrees that only women with normal healthy pregnancies should birth at home, but he believes that the excellent results he has had with home birth are partly due to lack of obstetrical interference. "Those familiar with home birth frequently observe that labors are shorter than average, more trouble free and more joyful to the mother. The babies are typically alert and more vigorous at birth, with excellent Apgar scores of nine or ten," he writes in *The Home Birth Book.*[5]

Holland has proven that where the system provides excellent prenatal care, childbirth education, trained nurse-midwives and a "mobile-unit" or "flying-squad" equipped for emergencies, home birth is a safe and healthy alternative to hospital birth. However, until this large scale organization occurs, I agree that there is an element of risk. As I mentioned in Chapter 1, the idea of an unprepared couple having an unattended home birth, as one couple who phoned me planned, makes me decidedly nervous. However, the use of the nurse-midwife in an informal, homey center, equipped adequately for complications, may be a workable alternative to home birth. I should add, though, that establishing such new centers is much more difficult and expensive than adding a "Lamaze Room" to an existing hospital.

Return of the Midwife

Essential to any backup system for home birth is the midwife, so beloved in Europe. In North America, the trend seems to be toward the trained nurse-midwife — a registered nurse who has completed additional education and clinical training in midwifery. In recent years, her services have been welcomed — not only for home birth, but to augment obstetrical care in the hospital birth.

But in most parts of the United States and Canada, midwives cannot legally attend home birth without a doctor's presence. The Campaign Association for the Legalization of Midwifery (CALM) and other groups are currently fighting for legal recognition of certified nurse-midwives. There are exceptions — in some inner-city areas and rural communities — where midwives are succesfully managing birth. For example, the Frontier Nursing Service, founded in 1925 in Kentucky, has delivered 20,000 babies. The Southeast Regional Council on Development of Nurse Midwifery, a six-state organization (Alabama, Florida, Louisiana, Mississippi, Georgia and South Carolina) trains nurse-midwives to handle total care for low-risk mothers, including delivery, at home or in hospital. And the Chicago Maternity Center, a medically directed home birth service with trained nurse-midwives and medical backup, performed more than 12,000 home births in Chicago from 1950 to 1960, without a single maternal mortality — at a time when the national incidence was two per 1,000.

Working with doctors, the midwife can inject a warm, personal touch into hospital obstetrics. Right now in Connecticut, about 20 certified nurse-midwives practice in conjunction with obstetricians. For normal pregnancies, these nurse-midwives handle regular checkups and prenatal care — taking time to discuss nutrition, infant care and related topics in a relaxed environment. Fathers may attend these sessions, which take place either at home or in a clinic.

According to Charlotte Houde, head of the Nurse-Midwife Education Program for Yale University, there is an increasing demand for new clinics and midwifery services across the United States.[6] Women who seek a more "sisterly" health care welcome the midwife — as do those women who appreciate the extended time and understanding she can provide. Not only can the nurse-midwife help make childbirth satisfying and safe, but — as in Holland — she can free the obstetrician to deal with complicated pregnancies.

Community Birth Center

The Maternity Center Association of New York was the first organization in North America to offer prenatal classes and also to open the first school of nurse midwifery in the United States. On October 9, 1975 the center opened its new "Childbearing Center", where women considered low-risk may give birth attended by trained nurse-midwives in a "home away from home" setting.

Set up to counteract the rise of home births with inadequate medical back-up, the center operates from a townhouse on East 92nd Street, a rather grand edifice which I visited some years ago when it was used as the office and headquarters of the Association.

The Childbearing Center provides prenatal care, childbirth education classes, infant and parenting programs as well as labor, delivery and post partum care. State licensed, it accepts for delivery only women with normal healthy pregnancies, and refers high risks to hospitals. To ensure continuity of care and preparation, it currently accepts as clients only women less than 20 weeks pregnant. Although it is equipped for regional anesthesia it is not equipped for general anesthesia or Caesarean births. The center, in addition to examining rooms and a classroom — including toys for other children accompanying their mothers on check-ups — has an early labor lounge. Women in early labor can relax here with their families or stroll in the garden.

The combination labor-delivery rooms here are of the same style as Manchester's except that a regular hospital bed is used for delivery. Women are given flexibility in birth position; unnecessary routines such as shaves, enemas and episiotomies are done only when absolutely necessary. The mother is given her baby immediately after birth; it is examined by a pediatrician before discharge and the family heads for home twelve hours later. Siblings may remain with their mother for the birth or be supervised in the child care room.

The medical team includes nurse-midwives, some trained in Holland and Britain, some U. S. trained, and obstetricians. Visiting nurses visit the woman at home on the first day and again on the third to fifth. By mid-July of 1976, the Center had done 44 births and had run into considerable opposition from both physicians and government. The non-profit association charges $750 per birth, considerably below the cost of a hospital delivery. In New York, charges for a "normal" birth routinely run as high as $3,000. The Center applied for and received permission to be reimbursed for services under the federally funded Medicaide assistance program, but the City of New York had, by late summer 1976, so far refused to grant them a vendor's licence necessary to allow their clients to use the plan.

Centres like this one seem to me to be a very real answer to the birth problem — but a lot of pioneer work with both government and the medical profession is needed before they come into wide use.

Conspiracy of Silence?

Unfortunately, the number of prepared (via prenatal classes) women we see you could count on one hand. Is that the fault of the nurses or the doctor?

— *Jinetta Oakes, R.N., caseroom nurse.*[7]

As a labor room nurse, I am shocked at the number of women who enter pregnancy and ultimately labor without so much as picking up a book to see what is

*happening to their bodies or what labor is all about and
how they can best cope with it.*

—K. Hammer.[8]

*I've had two children by means of an epidural while
my husband paced the waiting room — and both times I
felt cheated somehow but I didn't know why. During all
that time, nobody told me that I had a choice in the way
my baby would be born. It was only afterwards that a
friend was lucky enough to have PC and I learned what
I had missed.*

— Diana M.

Diana M.'s experience is typical of the majority of women
giving birth in North America today. As a guest on numerous
radio hotline shows, I've heard her words repeated countless
times: "Nobody told me I had a choice!" To me, it's incredible that an amazingly effective system of childbirth —
used by millions of women in the civilized world — is not so
much as *mentioned* when a woman goes to her obstetrician.
The woman I spoke with one afternoon in our park is another
typical example. While we watched our children play, the
conversation swung around to PC, and she was eager to
discuss it. She wished she had used it, she said — but her doctor, whom she adores, never discussed it during her four
pregnancies.

I agree with Jinetta Oakes that the shockingly low number
of prepared women is not the fault of the nurse. But I feel that
it is partly the fault of the doctor, or, more accurately, of the
medical training which has produced him or her. It is
significant that the majority of couples in my classes are sent
to me not by their doctors, but by friends who swear by this
method. When they tell their doctor what they are learning,
his response is usually benign tolerance — "Oh, yes, that's
nice" . . . "That can't do you any harm." In Montreal, there
are only fifteen doctors who routinely refer women to me and
are enthusiastic about the results — but usually only after the

woman herself initiates the topic.

The "conspiracy of silence" is rooted in medical school curriculae which focus on the managed birth — and either omit PC entirely or dismiss it as a fad for which very few women are suited. I've tried to find the conspirators. But I don't believe there are many professionals who are actively withholding information — just a lot of busy people unaware of the benefits of PC. The only villains I can find are the apathy and ignorance which have conspired to produce a lack of information about PC. But the resultant silence is the most effective sabotage I can imagine.

Ms. Hammer is shocked at the number of women who do not read about pregnancy and birth, and I agree that with so many books available on the subject, PC should be common knowledge. But not every woman will see these books. Every pregnant woman will see a doctor at regular intervals during pregnancy: if PC is not mentioned at these visits, who can blame her for assuming it is not important?

If we want to break the conspiracy of silence, education is a must. We can improve existing services and work towards ideals such as the labor-delivery room and the birth center. But the current system will not change greatly until all pregnant women and obstetrical personnel are educated in Prepared Childbirth. If we want our society to treat childbirth as a natural and normal human function rather than a mysterious medical event, we need a four-point system of education:

1. Community education.
2. Education of the existing obstetrical staff.
3. Education of trainee obstetrical staff.
4. Consumer information.

1. Community Education

Dr. Pierre Vellay refers to the negative attitudes surrounding childbirth, so prevalent in our society, as "psychological pollution". If we want to eliminate psychological pollution, we must educate children from pre-school up. We need to

transfer the idea to our children that childbirth is tremendously hard work but can be a satisfying experience for man
and woman. This concept should be reinforced in schools by
films dealing with birth appropriate to age group, carried
through to high school and college by films, discussion
groups and literature on birth preparation and parenting,
stressing the role of both parents. Incorporating such childbirth information in existing sex education programs would
be a positive beginning in the fight against psychological
pollution.

A pipe dream? Not really. I've seen the effects of such an
approach. There's a whole new group of parents who have
shared a prepared childbirth and who are conveying the joy of
their experience to their children. At my parents' "drop-in"
evenings, parents' older children frequently attend. They
listen to parents describe and discuss their births; they look at
the babies, and occasionally watch films. Some of the
children have photographs of their own births. One little boy
whose parents attended my classes seven years ago to prepare
for his birth brought "his" birth pictures in one night to show
a class. He was bursting with pride and hoped his parents
would take pictures of his baby brother or sister.

"Deirdre's favorite bedtime story is the story of how she
was born," my friend Jo Ann told me when her daughter was
two years old. "She likes to hear the part about Daddy
working very hard to hold me up. Sometimes I think she
believes Daddy worked harder than Mummy!"

My own daughter has watched classes for couples at our
home since she was born, has watched films and frequently
glances at her own birth photos. I overheard her talking to a
friend some time ago. The little girl's mother was expecting
her second child soon. Tilke told her matter of factly, "Your
mummy will push the baby out of her uterus", and she
promptly got down on the floor and went through the practice routine for pushing she watched one night at a class.

Positive information passed on from the parent is perhaps
the most valuable, but this should be followed up by

education for childbirth and parenting starting in pre-school, presented naturally and simply. I've spoken to groups of children about birth from time to time, showing pictures and discussing how the parents feel. They're fascinated, but take it perfectly in their stride. It's not a big deal. I've also spoken to high school and college students, and have been gratified by the interest of the male students — not just in anatomy and physiology but in feelings and sharing.

Recently I was a guest on yet another radio talk show about Prepared Childbirth. I was saddened by the calls: one unhappy woman after another phoned in to describe her birth experience. Most women had not known about childbirth education, but of the minority of women who had taken some sort of course, many had been frustrated by hospital staff in their attempts to use what was taught. Every caller had in some way been disappointed by her birth. This show convinced me of the unfortunate fact that most women are not prepared for childbirth — and that most hospitals are not prepared for the woman who is.

How One Community Is Changing:

When David and I founded the Montreal Childbirth Education Association, there was only one hospital in the city where evening classes for couples were provided, free; where flexibility in birth methods was relatively easy to arrange; where staff were usually familiar with Prepared Childbirth techniques; where fathers were uniformly welcome; and where breastfeeding, rooming in and sibling visiting were part of the total family-centred approach.

We started MCEA with a core of interested parents who had shared in the prepared births of their children, and a small group of interested professionals. We aimed to promote prepared childbirth in the community by:

1. Regular public meetings on subjects relating to pregnancy, childbirth and parenting.
2. Provision of a telephone information and referral service to give information about classes, doctors and hospitals.

3. Improving obstetrical care in the hospitals by workshops and meetings for hospital staff.

4. Printing a guidebook to childbirth education and related services in Montreal.

Attendance at the first meeting was 26. Within six months we had 500 to a meeting led by the pioneer of the Lamaze Method in North America, Elisabeth Bing. As part of a continual media campaign, David and I have done many radio and television shows, usually accompanied by prepared couples who talked about their experiences. Monthly meetings now average an attendance of several hundred, and more and more couples have asked for flexibility in the hospitals. Within a year of MCEA's founding, there were a dozen or so evening courses for couples in the city, and fathers were almost routinely participating in the birth.

Hundreds of our members and couples who have attended meetings have chosen their obstetricians thoughtfully. Many changed doctors when they found that the doctor's views were not couple oriented — first explaining to the doctors why they were changing. Many of those doctors paused to examine their attitudes and changed their former policies.

When the hospital stay proved rigid and hospital oriented instead of patient oriented, many of these couples discussed the situation with nurses, and followed by writing letters. They were well heard.

The MCEA is now four years old but the changes in the city are dramatic. Reports from my couples recently include the following:

> *Both the attending nurse and the doctor were very supportive and encouraging. I found the nurses helpful with breastfeeding . . .*
>
> *The staff were tremendously supportive, explained everything, offered the baby for nursing on the table and gave verbal support with breastfeeding . . .*
>
> *Hospital willing to fill your requests, but you must know what you want and ask for it . . .*

I found everyone extremely supportive . . .
The support was excellent when they saw I really was
prepared . . .

It is eventually you, the consumer of obstetrical care who
can change the system. And it *is* changing. In Montreal now,
most of my couples are getting exactly the sort of birth experience they'd like — often bypassing traditional hospital
routines. The MCEA has laid the groundwork here, and in
hundreds of cities other childbirth groups are also promoting
the trend to a less mechanized, more personal system of childbirth.

2. Existing Obstetrical Staff.

The Doctor. Although currently medical schools do not
teach the principles of Prepared Childbirth in anything but a
cursory way, doctors are changing and becoming supportive
of the method. The doctor who discusses PC with his clients
and who watches their satisfaction in labor becomes a convert. In turn he refers more women and their mates to classes,
and more classes begin to meet the demand.

The doctor's office has tremendous potential for
education. I've sat in doctor's offices where the only reading
material was a tattered series of outdated magazines which
one would never read unless driven by extreme boredom. But,
in the Manchester clinic where Drs. Sumner, Wheeler and
Smith practice, the waiting rooms are a whole mini-course in
childbirth education. Clients can browse through the latest
books on pregnancy, birth and parenting; and pamphlets
about Prepared Childbirth, breastfeeding information, etc. —
not to mention a whole set of video tapes about childbirth and
parenting, which they can watch on the spot!

Almost every woman spends hours sitting in clinic and office waiting rooms — this time can be useful. When I taught
at the Catherine Booth Hospital in Montreal, two mornings a
week were obstetrical clinic time, with up to forty women
waiting in an auditorium. Coffee was served and I talked in-

formally about nutrition, preparation for birth, labor and the post partum period, taking small groups of women to the mats at the back of the room for short exercise periods and preparation for birth techniques. Other children would watch their mothers, friends or fathers coached and the nurses in the examining rooms handed out booklets about birth and baby care. This on-the-spot education proved extremely effective and reached many women who — because of other children, babysitting and transport problems — could not attend a series of classes. One summer a public health nurse and I held drop-in classes in the kitchen of a community centre. Women and their families crowded in to watch films and discuss birth. That also was on-the-spot education.

Many doctors have all sorts of misunderstandings about Prepared Childbirth and what it is that couples ask for. I spoke at obstetrical Grand Rounds at a large general hospital some time ago. A number of the doctors present still associated Prepared Childbirth with ''natural'' or non-medicated childbirth, and viewed any childbirth education as a movement in which women would refuse the benefits of modern obstetrics for some unclear, misguidedly idealistic principle. One doctor was concerned that childbirth education did not deal with complications. He believed that when Caesareans or forceps were needed women became depressed because they had been led to believe that their birth would be a normal vaginal one. I explained that classes should prepare a woman for any kind of birth; that preparation only for a simple vaginal delivery was poor preparation. The couple who accompanied me and brought their baby along talked about their birth and expectations. I think that meeting, and many like it which I have had with medical people, cleared up a number of common misconceptions.

The Nurse. Obstetrical nurses base their attitudes in accordance with the numbers of prepared women they see. At hospitals where the prepared woman is a rarity, nursing care is usually geared to the unprepared woman: routines which center around the medicated birth dominate. Many maternity nurses trained at a time when very little attention was given to psychoprophylaxis: unless in-service education programs are provided, such a nurse may have little opportunity to become familiar with Prepared Childbirth. I have observed that most of the "hospital hassles" with nurses are the result of misunderstanding what the prepared couple are doing.

Many hospitals are now realizing there is a great need for regular in-service education. In the last few years I have spoken many times to hospital staff about Prepared Childbirth and couples' expectations. Some time ago I was invited to speak to a group of more than a hundred obstetrical nurses from Montreal and surrounding areas. I showed slides of births I had filmed in Holland: the initial reaction to labor-delivery room, no stirrups, no "prep" was at first surprise but then approval. A number of nurses came up after the talk and wanted more detail of a "non-managed" birth. In the following months, I found nurses who had listened to the talk much more supportive of my couples than they had been previously — and many changes were made in Montreal hospitals.

3. Trainee Medical Personnel

Many nursing schools are now spending a good deal of time teaching the principles of family-centred maternity care, and usually attention is given to Prepared Childbirth techniques. I believe that as these students graduate, they are putting into effect the hospital changes necessary for flexible and supportive couple-oriented childbirth.

I frequently speak to student nurses: many of them attend the MCEA public meetings and I've found them enthusiastic about P.C. Each week, student nurses and physiotherapists attend my classes, watching and talking with the pregnant couples, and listening to new parents discuss their birth experiences. These students are learning as much from the couples as from any formal instruction.

Since 1974, I have co-ordinated and taught the undergraduate obstetrical program to physiotherapists at McGill University. The program is essentially in psychoprophylaxis, with opportunity for students to talk with prepared couples about their experiences. Soon the effects of this program will be noticeable, and as one student told me, "It will influence my attitudes to birth when I have a child".

4. Consumer Information

One of my initial ideas in the early days of MCEA was to print a booklet which would give newcomers to the city help in choosing a doctor, hospital, course, etc. In 1974, David and I compiled such a guidebook, the printing made possible by a grant from IBM of Canada, under a program to encourage employee participation in the community. (The employee in this case was Austin Down, an enthusiastic member of the MCEA committee.)

The information we included was a brief 48 page version of the "How to Choose . . ." sections given in more detail in this book, plus the detailed questionnaire to Montreal doctors I've mentioned in Chapter 5, as well as a guide to day care facilities in Montreal, nutrition and breastfeeding information, services for the single mother and other community services relating to childbirth and parenting. Our *Guide to childbirth education and related services in Montreal* was a headache to produce. Even with volunteers working on surveys and other details, David and I spent a long, hot summer laboring on the booklet in our "spare time" which usually turned out to be the small hours of the morning — but the results were certainly worth all the effort. We have distributed it free through doctors' offices, clinics, day care centres, women's groups, colleges and our public meetings. It has been a strong factor in producing change in the community and has influenced many doctors and hospitals to change in a very short time. I'd recommend the idea to other groups, in spite of the work involved; in fact, we have had requests for the guide by many other North American groups who are considering a similar plan.

One aspect of childbirth which I have not gone into in this book is *cost*. All women have, I believe, the right to a low-cost birth. This is available in Canada under a federally run Medicare program, and is provided in many other countries, although currently birth in the United States may run to several thousand dollars. Recently I spoke to a friend in Vermont, who has just given birth to her second baby. I asked how much it cost and she replied "Oh, about $1,000" — even though she had returned home with her daughter after a brief two-day hospital stay! An itemized account of birth cost shows anesthesia rating high on the list. ($100 or more, depending on the hospital, is a conservative estimate.)

The province of Quebec is currently moving towards a government run peri-natal program. In moving into the prenatal education field in this way, the government rightly senses that there is money to be saved here. If the number of births where anesthesia is used could be cut in half, any universal childbirth education program would more than pay for itself in dollar terms, as well as reducing human suffering. One possibility in this area might be a blend of the socialist and free enterprise approach to childbirth education, with government funding on a fee-for-service basis to childbirth educators similar to the plan for physicians under the Canadian Medicare system.

However, not even widespread childbirth preparation classes will change our maternity system until every obstetrical consumer demands change. It is to the advantage of our entire society that babies be born not only as healthy as possible, but into families as loving as possible. Close bonding of parent-child and parent-parent is, I believe, impaired by our current maternity system.

In recent years, sociologists have lamented the breakdown of both the institution of marriage and the family unit. One in every three marriages in North America ends in divorce — a frightening statistic if you happen to be a young man or woman in love and considering marriage. The oft-cited breakdown in parent-child communications is equally frightening if you happen to be a man or woman contemplating, or in the process of having, a baby.

I would never suggest that a couple have a baby in order to save a sagging marriage. (Far from it! I would advise them to stay childfree and seek marriage counselling). But I have observed that childbirth education classes combined with shared birth and parenting seem to increase a couple's chances for a healthy marriage and a strong family life. Out of the four thousand couples I have prepared for birth — hundreds of whom I have kept in contact with — to my knowledge, only one marriage has ended in divorce. A statistician might object that possibly only couples with successful marriages would be attracted to shared childbirth. But the couples I see in my classes represent a cross-section of the whole gamut of marital relations. They share one thing in common, however: during the nine-month stretch in which they attend my classes, I nearly always notice a definite change in their attitudes toward each other. In both the most loving of couples and those who previously appeared strained with each other, I note increased intimacy and a growing sense of appreciation towards the mate.

Rachel and Morgan were among the "strained" group. They attended my classes to prepare for their second child — and I nearly expected them to be divorced by the time the child was born. Morgan was reluctant to attend classes. For the first birth, he had attended one or two prenatal classes where the father was included as a spectator — but no attempt had been made to involve him as a participant. Rachel had equal reservations about my class — attending only on the strong recommendation of both her best friend and her obstetrician.

During early classes, Rachel kept putting Morgan down, describing in detail how he had been no help at all the first time around. He had been in the labor room with her. As contractions grew stronger, Rachel told him he bothered her, and both were relieved when he chose to remain in the waiting room where his son was born. But as classes progressed, I watched Morgan change from an uneasy, uninterested observer to an enthusiastic member of the group. He began to express his opinions quite forcefully, much to the surprise of Rachel, who looked at him with new respect.

After their baby, Benjy, was born, they came back as the guest family, with their two sons — Morgan nonchalantly carrying the baby in a front pack. They talked about the birth. Rachel had had a somewhat long and hard labor. "She was amazing", Morgan told the group. "She got a little cranky during transition, of course — but nothing like the last time around." Then he added the cliché I hear from almost every prepared father. "I felt *needed*."

"I couldn't have done it without him," Rachel said. "Toward the end, I became very muddled and the staff were too busy to give me much attention. But Morgan encouraged me and worked with me through every single contraction, so that I never felt out of control . . . and he's so good with Benjy!"

Five years later, a man phoned me and identified himself as a friend of Morgan's. He wanted to enrol with his wife. "Morgan says your classes saved their marriage", he said frankly. "This is our second baby, too, and I think we need all the help we can get!"

It seems to me that an ounce of prophylaxis is worth a pound of cure. Across North America, billions of dollars are spent each year on marriage and family counselling — working with unhappy adults and their children. Perhaps not every case of a battered baby, juvenile delinquent or marriage breakup can be prevented by shared, non-interfered-with childbirth, and preparation for the demanding role of parent. But I believe that a good start can provide a firm basis for a happy family that can withstand the stress of modern living. A society is as healthy as its basic unit — the family — and it is in the interest of every member of the community that healthy babies be born into healthy families. In this respect, each baby born is everybody's baby!

Consumerism popularized the trend to a childbirth made as

painless as possible by medical intervention. By the millions, women welcomed drugs and the managed birth — in ignorance of both the possible side-effects and the existence of another method of achieving the goal of childbirth without suffering. Today, however, more and more consumers are questioning the need for massive technological intrusion into everyday living. The term "quality of life" has become a household word while humanity, approaching the twenty-first century, searches for the small and personal in a frighteningly complex and mechanized environment. That childbirth is receiving such close scrutiny is not surprising. Change is inevitable if you, the consumer, insist on your rights.

A joyous, loving birth may be only the beginning, but it's a crucial first step.

Glossary

Amniotic fluid (am-ni-ot'ic): water-like fluid contained in the membranous sac ("bag of waters") surrounding the fetus. It helps to support the fetus, permits it to move, prevents loss of heat and absorbs shocks.

Analgesic (an'al-ge'sic): drug which relieves pain without causing unconsciousness.

Anesthetic: agent used to induce loss of feeling with or without loss of consciousness.

Apgar score: a scale developed by the late Virginia Apgar, which rates the newborn baby by observation of color, muscle tone, pulse, reflex irritibility and respiration. Usually given at one minute, five minutes and thirty minutes after birth.

Braxton-Hicks Contractions: intermittent contractions of the uterus. Increasingly noticeable in late pregnancy as the uterus prepares itself for labor.

Breech: delivery of the baby with buttocks or legs first.

Caesarean or cesarean section: operation by which the baby is removed from the uterus by cutting through the abdominal wall. According to legend, Julius Caesar was born this way.

Cervix (ser'vix): the necklike, narrow opening of the uterus.

Colostrum (Ko'los-trum): the nutritious, clear, yellowish substance produced by the breasts for the baby before the actual milk comes in.

"Complete": refers to dilation of the cervix. A woman is said to be "complete" when the cervix is sufficiently dilated for the baby to pass through — usually 10 cm. or five fingers. (One finger = 2 cm.)

Contraction: tightening and shortening of the uterine muscles during labor, causing effacement and dilatation of the cervix, and contributing to the outward descent of the baby.

Crowning: appearance of the presenting part of baby at perineum during second stage.

Dilatation (dil'a-ta'tion): gradual opening and drawing up of the cervix to permit passage of the baby. Progress is measured by estimating the diameter of the opening cervix in fingers or cm.

Effacement: thinning of the cervix, which may occur in early labor or the last few weeks of pregnancy.

Effleurage (ef-ler-azhe'): light rhythmic massage — done over lower abdomen during the labor in Lamaze Method.

Engagement: means that the presenting part of the baby has moved into the upper opening (inlet) of the pelvic canal and is in its beginning position for birth. May be noticed by the mother as "lightening". Baby is sometimes said to have "dropped". Mother's breathing usually becomes easier after engagement.

Epidural (ep'i-du'ral): regional anesthesia introduced into the extradural space in the lower back. It blocks the passage of sensory nerve impulses to the brain, but does not affect consciousness.

Episiotomy (e-pi'si-ot'o-my): an incision made into the perineum between the vaginal opening and anus prior to birth, to facilitate delivery of the baby.

False labor: regular or irregular contractions of the uterus strong enough to be interpreted as true labor — but with no dilating effect on the cervix.

Fetus: scientific term for baby from the end of the third month of pregnancy until delivery.

First stage of labor: the period of labor when the cervical opening effaces and dilates to let the baby pass through. It is the longest part of labor (90% of the total duration) and ends when the woman is "complete".

Induction: initiating labor by the use of medication (an oxytocic). Usually given intravenously.

"I.V.": hospital slang for the intravenous procedure — in which a sterile fluid is dripped into the vein for the purpose of nutrition, hydration, or medication.

Lamaze Method (la-mahz'): the Russian psychoprophylactic method, in the form adapted by French obstetrician Fernand Lamaze.

Lithotomy position (li-thot'-a-my): delivery position in which the woman lies on her back, her legs supported by stirrups.

Lochia (lo'chi-a): discharge of blood, mucus and tissue from the uterus after the birth of the baby. May continue several weeks and vary in amount.

Molding: the shaping of the baby's head to adjust itself to the size and shape of the birth canal.

Monitrice: a female instructor who coaches the woman through childbirth — usually using psychoprophylaxis. Introduced first in France by Lamaze.

Mucus plug: a plug of heavy mucus which blocks the cervical canal during preg-

nancy.

Multipara (mul-tip'a-ra): a woman who has had a previous birth. "Multip" is hospital slang.

Natural Childbirth: a term coined by British physician Grantly Dick-Read, to described an educated birth unobstructed by fear and the resulting tension and pain — thus minimizing the need for medication. Often misinterpreted as simply childbirth without drugs, primitive childbirth, or instinctive childbirth; or confused with Prepared Childbirth, "Lamaze", or psychoprophylaxis.

Neuromuscular Control: the ability to consciously make your muscles do what you want them to do. Synonyms: Complete Release, Controlled Release, Controlled Relaxation. Stressed in Prepared Childbirth.

Oxytoxic: drug used to stimulate uterine contractions. Useful in starting or aiding labor. Given by injection routinely after birth.

Pelvic floor: an interrelated muscle group forming support for the rectum, urethra, bladder and internal reproductive organs.

Pelvis: the bony ring which joins the spine and legs. Its central opening forms the walls of the birth canal.

Perinatal (per'i-na'tal): relating to birth.

Perineum (per'i-ne'um): external tissues surrounding the anus and vulva.

"Pit Drip": hospital slang for intravenous solution containing pitocin, an oxytoxic, used to stimulate or induce labor.

Placenta (pla-cen'ta): the vascular structure developed in pregnancy through which nutrition, excretion and respiration take place between mother and baby. Also called "afterbirth".

Post partum: after giving birth.

Prenatal: before giving birth.

Prepared Childbirth (PC): An approach to childbirth, which prepares the woman physically, emotionally and psychologically to participate actively in labor, usually with the support of a coach — in most cases, the baby's father. PC stresses *learned* rather than "natural" responses, the term is often used interchangeably with PPM and the Lamaze Method; other variations include the Kitzinger, Wright and Bradley approaches.

Primipara (pri-mip'-a-ra): woman having her first baby. "Primip" is hospital slang.

Psychoprophylaxis and PPM (si'ko-pro'fi-lak'sis): The word "psychoprophylaxis" literally means "mind prevention of pain". The psychopro-

phylactic method (PPM) originated in Russia, based on the work of Pavlov. By means of the conditioned reflex, the woman is prepared during pregnancy to work actively with the changing sensations of labor — thus minimizing pain, and giving her a controlling role in childbirth.

Ripe: a word used to describe the softened condition of the cervix when it is ready for the onset of labor.

Second stage of labor: the period of time when the baby passes from the uterus through the vagina and is born. Can last from a few minutes to several hours.

"Show": the reddish-colored mucus which sometimes announces the onset of labor or is gradually discharged during labor. It represents the sloughing off of the protective mucus plug. (This is blood-streaked or tinged mucus — not bleeding.)

Stimulation of labor: Surgical rupture of membranes or administration of an oxytoxic medicine after labor has started. (Enemas are sometimes used this way).

"Term": completed cycle of pregnancy. Near due-date, the pregnant woman is said to be "at term".

Third stage of labor: the period of time after the baby is born until the time when the placenta has separated and is expelled. Usually lasts from one to twenty minutes. (Also known as "placental stage".)

Transition: The end of the first stage, from about 6-7 to 10 cm. dilation. Most active phase of labor.

Ultra-Prepared Childbirth (UPC): My own method of intensive PC for the couple, which adds to psychoprophylaxis the techniques of communication and assertiveness — necessary to ensure freedom of choice in the hospital setting.

Uterus: muscular, pear-shaped organ of gestation: consists of a fundus and a narrower lower portion called the cervix. Also called "womb".

Vagina: the curved, elastic, birth canal, five or six inches long, from the vulva to the cervix.

Vernix caseosa (ver'nix ca'se-o'sa): protective white material, cheese-like in consistency, covering the skin of the newborn. This "baby cold cream" is seen in varying amounts.

Vulva (vul'va): the external female reproductive organs, generally understood as the external lips or folds outside the vaginal entrance.

Footnotes

Chapter 1

1. Doris Haire, *The Cultural Warping of Childbirth,* A Special Report for the International Childbirth Education Association, 1972, p. 5.
2. North American figures are the result of the author's research and correspondence with childbirth educators. Dutch figures were supplied by the obstetrical unit at the University Hospital and the Wilhemina Gasthuis, Amsterdam in 1975.

Chapter 3

1. R. Burchell, "Predelivery Removal of Fubic Hair", *Obstet. and Gynec.,* 1964, 24:272-273; H. Kantor et al., "Value of Shaving the Pudendal-Perineal Area. . ." *Obstet and Gynec.,* 1965, 25:509-512. Both quoted by Haire.
2. Roberto Caldeyro-Barcia, "Some Consequences of Obstetrical Interference", *Birth and the Family Journal,* Spring, 1975, Vol. 2:34-36.
3. Madeleine Shearer, "Some Deterrents to Objective Evaluation of Fetal Monitors", *ibid.,* p. 58.
4. Stewart E. Taylor, "Editorial", *Obstet. Gynec, Survey,* June, 1974.
5. Shearer, *op. cit.,* p. 59.
6. Charles E. McLennan and Eugene C. Sandberg, *Synopsis of Obstetrics,* St. Louis, C.V. Mosby, 1974, p. 466.
7. K.S. Koh et al, "Experience with Fetal Monitoring. . ." *Obstet. Gynec. Survey,* Sept. 1975, p. 596. See also Haverkamp, A.D., Thomson, H.E., McFee, J.G., and Cetrulo, C., "The Evaluation of Continuous Fetal Heart Rate Functioning in High Risk Pregnancy", *Am. J. Ob. Gyn.,* 125:310-320; and Banta, H. David, Thacker, Stephen B., National Center for Health Services Research publication, Dec. 3, 1978.
8. Haire, p. 58.
9. L.B. Altstatt., "Transplacental hyponatremia in the newborn infant", *Journal of Pediatrics,* 1965: pp. 985-988. F. Battaglia et al, "Fetal blood studies, XIII. . ." *Pediatrics,* 1960, 25:2-10.
9a. Ronald Myers, "Brain damage not caused by lack of oxygen", *Medical Post,* March, 1977.
10. Sandberg and McLennan, p. 447.
11. Noel De Garis, "More Risks With Nine-to-Five Birth," *The Age,* Melbourne, Australia, Aug. 27, 1974.
12. Caldeyro-Barcia, p. 37. See also R.A. Cole et al, "Elective Induction of Labour", *Lancet,* May 1975, 1 (7915):1088; and Liston and Campbell, "Dangers of oxytocin-induced labor to fetuses", *Brit. Med. J.,* 1974, 3:606.
   As a result of hearings conducted by the FDA and U.S. Senate Committees relating to health, the labels on oxytocins now by law, carry a warning to the medical profession. The new labels urge caution in the use of oxytocin in medically indicated induction and augmentation of

labor. Wunderlich, Cherry, "Oxytoxic Labelling Requirements Implemented, *ICEA News,* 1978, 17:3-4.
13. Robert A. Bradley, Interview with Jay and Margie Hathaway for *American Academy of Husband-Coached Childbirth* (pamphlet).
14. As quoted by Deborah Tanzer, *Why Natural Childbirth,* New York, Doubleday, 1972, p. 43.
15. Tanzer, p. 47, also Lester B. Hazell, *Commonsense Childbirth,* New York, Berkley Windhover, 1969, 1976, p. 12.
16. Odile M. Plantevin, *Analgesia and Anaesthesia in Obstetrics,* Great Britain, Butterworths, 1973, p. 54.
17. Sumner J. Yaffe, "A clinical look at the problem of drugs in pregnancy. . ." *Canadian Medical Association J.* March, 1975, 1112:6:730. See also Y. Brackbill et al, "Obstetric premedication and infant outcome," *Am. J. Obstet. Gynec.,* 1974, 118:377.
18. T. Berry Brazelton, "What Childbirth Drugs Can Do to Your Child", *Redbook,* Feb. 1971, p. 65.
19. N.J. Eastman, "Editorial", *Obstet. Gynec. Survey,* 1962, 17:459-500.
20. H.R. Gordon, "Fetal brachycardia after paracervical block. . ." *New Eng. J. of Med.,* 1968, 279:910-914.
21. Plantevin, pp 121-124.
22. Koh, p. 13.
23. Burns and Gurtner, "Oxygen Transport. . .", *Johns Hopkins Mag,* March, 1976, pp. 18-22.
24. K. Standley et al. "Local-regional anesthesia during childbirth. . ." *Science,* Nov. 15, 1964, 86 (4164): 634-5.
25. E. Tronick et al, "Regional obstetric anaesthesia and newborn behavior. . ." *Pediatrics,* July, 1976, pp. 94-100. As quoted by Haire, p. 17.
26. Haire, p. 13.
27. Haire, p. 36.
28. Niles Newton, "The Effects of Disturbance on Labor", *Amer. J. Obstet. and Gynec.,* 1968, 101:1096-1102. R.E. Myers, "Maternal psychological stress and fetal asphyxia. . ." *Am. J. Obstet. and Gynec.,* 1 May, 1975, pp. 47-60.
29. Caldeyro-Barcia, p. 28. See also Humphrey, "A decrease in fetal pH. . . in the dorsal position", *Obstet. and Gynec. Br. Commonwealth,* Aug., 1974, pp. 600-2.
    Caldeyro-Barcia's latest studies conclude that in normal, spontaneous labors, the vertical position facilitates the progress of labor, shortens its duration and reduces maternal discomfort and pain. Caldeyro-Barcia, Roberto, "The Influence of Maternal Position During the Second Stage of Labor": address given to the Tenth Biennial Convention of the International Childbirth Education Association, 1978.
30. Chloe Fisher, "The Management of Labor", *Episiotomy — physical and emotional aspects,* Britain, National Childbirth Trust, p. 9.
31. N. Butler, "A national long term study of perinatal hazards", Sixth World Congress, Fed. Int'l, Gynec and Obstet., 1970; quoted by Haire, p. 24.

32. Sheila Kitzinger, "Emotional aspects of episiotomy and postnatal sexual adjustment", *Episiotomy — physical and emotional aspects,* op. cit., p. 18.
33. Diony Young, "Cesarean in the United States: a Sobering Situation", *ICEA News,* November, 1979; 18:4.
34. Banta-Thacker.

Chapter 5
1. Merrill, B.S., and Gibbs, C.E. "Planned Vaginal Delivery Following Cesarean Section", *Obstet. Gyn.* 1973, 42:589.

Chapter 6
1. Ashley Montagu, *Life Before Birth,* London, Longmans, 1961, p. 22.
2. Montagu, pp. 26-28.
3. Montagu, p. 25. See also Agnes Higgins et al, "Preliminary Report of a Nutrition Study. . ." *Canadian J. Dietetics Assn,* 1971, 37:1:17: and N.J. Eastman and E. Jackson, "Weight relationships in pregnancy. . ." *Obstet-Gynec, Survey,* 1968, 23:1003-1025.
4. Montagu, pp. 26-28; also B.S. Burke, "Nutrition and its relation to the complications of pregnancy. . ." *Amer. J. Pub. Health,* 1945, 35:334.
5. Haire, postscript.
   The Preventibility of Perinatal Injury, published by the National Foundation of the U.S. March of Dimes, 1974.
6. Lynn Dallin, *The Pregnant Woman's Low Calorie Cookbook,* New York, Doubleday, 1969 (foreword).
7. André B. Lalonde, Unpublished paper, *Nutrition in Maternal health Care,* Montreal, 1975.
8. T.H. Brewer, "Pregnant — and want your child?" *Nutrition Action Group* (pamphlet), San Francisco.
9. Montagu, pp. 90-92, 92-97.
   H. Van Vunakis et al, "Nicotine. . .in the second trimester of pregnancy", *Am. J. Obstet. Gynec.,* Sept, 1974, pp. 64-66. D. Rush, "Examination of the relationship between birthweight, cigarette smoking during pregnancy. . ." *J. Obstet. Gyn. Br. Commonwealth,* Oct., 1974, pp. 746-52.
10. Yaffe, p. 733.
11. Haire (postscript).
12. "DES seen threat to sons of women who took it", *Ottawa Journal,* Dec. 10, 1975.
13. Yaffe, p. 729.
14. Yaffe, p. 729.
15. "Tranquilizers linked to birth defects", *Ottawa Journal,* August, 1976.
16. Mortimer G. Rosen and Lynn Rosen, *Your Baby's Brain Before Birth,* New York, Plume Books, 1975, p. 56. Yaffe, p. 730.
17. Haire (postscript).
18. Haire (postscript).
19. Yaffe, p. 733.

Chapter 7

1. Karma and Michael Donnelly, *Husband-Wife Teaching Teams in Childbirth Education,* Madison, Wisconsin, Parentcraft, 1973, pp. 1-2.
2. Particularly applicable to the woman in childbirth are the following clauses of the Patient's Bill of Rights:

    (1)   The patient has a right to considerate and respectful care.

    (2)   The patient has the right to obtain from his physician complete current information concerning his diagnosis, treatment and prognosis in terms the patient can reasonably be expected to understand. . .

    (3)   The patient has the right to receive from his physician information necessary to give informed consent prior to the start of any procedure and/or treatment. . .

    (4)   The patient has the right to refuse treatment to the extent permitted by law, and to be informed of the medical consequences of his action.

    (5)   The patient has the right to every consideration of his privacy concerning his own medical care program. Case discussion, consultation, examination and treatment are confidential and should be conducted discreetly. Those not directly involved in his care must have permission of the patient to be present.

    (6)   The patient has the right to expect that all communications and records pertaining to his care should be treated as confidential. . .

    (9)   The patient has the right to be advised if the hospital proposes to engage in or perform human experimentation affecting his care or treatment. The patient has the right to refuse to participate in such research projects. . .

    (12) The patient has the right to know what hospital rules and regulations apply to his conduct as a patient.

Chapter 8

1. Stephanie Caruna, "Childbirth for the joy of it", *Playgirl,* March, 1974.
2. Tanzer, p. 162.
3. Murray W. Enkin, "Family Centred Maternity Care", *Canadian Family Physician,* April, 1973, p. 48.
4. *Husbands in the Delivery Room,* ICEA pamphlet, 1965, reprinted 1971, p. 16.
5. *Ibid,* p. 25.
6. Margaret Mead, *Male and Female,* New York, Morrow, 1949, p. 238.
7. Margaret Mead, *Growing Up in New Guinea,* New York, Mentor, 1953, pp. 39, 49.
8. As quoted by Tanzer, p. 206.
9. Tanzer, p. 208.
10. Mead, *Male and Female,* p. 192.
11. Pamela Mason, *Marriage is the First Step to Divorce,* New York, Paul S. Eriksson, Inc., 1968, pp. 115-116.
12. Richard Flaste, "Where Expectant Fathers Deliver Their Own Babies", *New York Times,* August 8, 1975.
13. "A Family Affair", *Ms.,* May, 1973, p. 115.

THE RIGHTS OF THE PREGNANT PARENT

14. George J. Annas, "Childbirth and the Courts . . .", *Medicolegal News,* Spring, 1976, pp. 4-5.

Chapter 9

1. Plantevin, p. 22.

Chapter 10

1. Lee Salk, *Preparing for Parenthood,* New York, David McKay Co., 1974, p. 80.
2. Marshall H. Klaus, "Maternal Attachment: Importance of the first post partum days", *New England J. of Med.,* 286:9: 460-463. M. Klaus, J.H. Kennell et al. "Human Maternal behavior at the first contact with her young, *Pediatrics* 46: 187-192, 1970.
3. "Contact and IQ Linked", *Ottawa Journal,* June 22, 1976.
4. Pilar Farnsworth, *Birth* (pamphlet), Maryland, 1973.
5. Mabel Liddiard, *The Mothercraft Manual,* London, J. and A. Churchill Ltd., 1923 (10th ed., 1944) p. 45.
6. "M.D. Urges Breastfeeding", *Montreal Star,* May 19, 1976.
7. *Prenatal Care,* United States Department of Labor, Children's Bureau, 1930, p. 43.
8. J.W. Gerrard, "Breast-feeding: second thoughts", *Pediatrics,* Dec. 1974, pp. 757-64.
9. M. Robinson, "Infant Morbidity and Mortality . . ." *Lancet,* 260:788; H. Hodes, "Colustrum: A Valuable Source of Antibodies", *Ob-Gyn. Observer,* 1964, 3:7. Both quoted by Haire, p. 14.
   D.B. Jeliffe et al, "Human milk, nutrition and the world resource crisis", *Science,* May 9, 1975, pp. 557-61.
   F. Monckeberg, *Symposium of 9th International Congress of Nutrition,* Mexico City, 1973.
   Marvin S. Eiger and Sally Wendkos Olds, *The Complete Book* of Breastfeeding, New York, Bantam, 1973, p. 17.
10. B. Hall, "Changing Composition of Human Milk and Early Development . . ." *Lancet,* April, 1975, pp. 779-81. Eiger and Olds, p. 105.
11. J.I. Rodale, *Natural Health and Pregnancy,* New York, Pyramid Publications, 1968, pp. 252-254.
    J. Glaser, "The Dietary Prophylaxis of Allergic Diseases in Infancy," *J. Asthma Research,* 1966, 3:199-208.
12. Rodale, pp. 255-256.
    P. Frogatt et al, "Epidemiology of Sudden Unexpected Deaths in Infants . . ." *Brit. J. Prev. Soc. Med.,* 1971, 25:110-134.
    A. Bergman et al, "Sudden Infant Death Syndrome", *2nd Int'l Conf. Sudden Death in Infants,* U. of Washington Press, Seattle, 1970.
13. G. Tank, "Relation of Diet to Variation of Dental Caries", *J. Amer. Dental Ass'n,* 1965, 70:394-403. T. Graber, "Malocclusion: Extrinsic or General Factors", *Orthodontics: Principles and Practice,* Philadelphia,

Saunders Co., 1972. Both quoted by Haire, p. 14. Rodale, 206, 213.
14. Eiger and Olds, p. 7.
15. J.M. Shane and F. Naftolin, "Effect of Ergonovine Maleate on Puerperal Prolactin", *Am. J. Obstet. Gynec.,* Sept, 1974, pp. 129-31.
J.A. Clemens et al, "Inhibition of Prolactin Secretion . . ." *Endocrinology,* April, 1974, pp. 1171-6.
Cassady et al, "Ergot alkaloids . . . as inhibitors of prolactin release", *J. Med. Chem.,* March, 1974, pp. 300-7.
16. Mead, *Male and Female,* p. 270.

Chapter 12

1. Philip. Sumner, John P. Wheeler, Samuel G. Smith, "The Labor-Delivery Bed — Simplified Obstetrics", *Journal of Reproductive Medicine,* October, 1974, p. 4.
2. Philip Hager, "California Crackdown on Illegal Midwifery", *Los Angeles Times,* reprinted in the *Montreal Star,* June 12, 1974.
3. "MDs urged not to back mothers having babies at home", *Toronto Globe and Mail* (CP), August 25, 1976.
4. "Study Finds Home Beats Hospital", *Montreal Gazette,* November 20, 1975.
5. Russel J. Bunai, "A Pediatricians Point of View", *The Home Birth Book,* Washington, D. C., Inscape Corp., 1976, p. 56.
6. "U.S. trend sees midwives aid mothers-to-be", *Montreal Star* (AP), August, 1976.
7. A letter to the editor, *Homemaker's Magazine* (Toronto), Sept., 1975, p. 50, referring to the article by Carroll Allen, "Let's put the joy and dignity back into birthing," May, 1975, p. 18.
8. Same as above, p. 52.

Bibliography

Arms, Suzanne. *Immaculate Deception.* Boston: San Francisco Book Company/Houghton Mifflin Company, 1975.
*Bing, Elisabeth. *Six Practical Lessons for an Easier Birth.* New York: Harper and Row, 1965.
*Bradley, Robert A. *Husband-Coached Childbirth.* New York: Harper and Row, 1965.
Bowes, Watson A. Jr. Brackbille, Yvonne. Conway, Esther. Steinschneider, Alfred. *Monographs of the Society for Research and Child Development.* Chicago: University of Chicago Press, 1970.
Dick-Read, Grantly. *Childbirth Without Fear.* London: Whitefriars Press Ltd., 1942.
Ehrenreich, Barbara. English, Deirdre. *Witches, Midwives and*

286 THE RIGHTS OF THE PREGNANT PARENT

Nurses: A history of women healers. (Old Westbury, N.Y.): Feminist Press, 2nd ed., 1973. Glass Mountain Pamplet no. 1.

*Eiger, Marvin S. Olds, Sally Wendkos. *The Complete Book of Breastfeeding.* New York: Bantam Books, 1973.

Haire, Doris. *The Cultural Warping of Childbirth.* A Special Report by the International Childbirth Education Association, 1972.

*Hazell, Lester. *Commonsense Childbirth.* New York: Berkley Windhover, 1969, 1976.

Heardman, Helen. *A Way to Natural Childbirth.* Edinburgh: E and S. Livingstone, 1949.

*Karmel, Marjorie. *Thank You, Dr. Lamaze.* New York: Lippincott, 1959.

Kitzinger, Sheila. *Episiotomy — Physical and Emotional Aspects.* London: National Childbirth Trust,

*Lamaze, Fernand. *Painless Childbirth.* London: Burke, 1958.

*Leboyer, Frederick. *Birth Without Violence.* New York: Alfred Knopf, 1975.

Liddiard, Mabel. *The Mothercraft Manual.* London: J. and A. Churchill Ltd., 1944 (10th edition).

McLennan, Charles E. Sandberg, Eugene C. *Synopsis of Obstetrics.* St. Louis: C.V. Mosby Co., 9th ed. 1974.

Mead, Margaret. *Male and Female.* New York: Morrow, 1949. *Growing Up in New Guinea.* New York: Mentor, 1953.

*Milinaire, Caterine. *Birth.* New York: Harmony Books, 1974.

*Montagu, Ashley. *Life Before Birth.* London: Longmans, 1964. *Touching.* New York: Perennial Library, Columbia University Press, 1971.

Plantevin, Odile M. *Analgesia and Anaesthesia in Obstetrics.* London: Butterworths, 1973.

*Pryor, Karen. *Nursing Your Baby.* New York: Harper and Row, 1963.

Rodale, J.I. *Natural Health and Pregnancy.* New York: Pyramid Books, 1968.

Rosen, Mortimer G. Rosen, Lynn. *Your Baby's Brain Before Birth.* New York: Plume Book 1975.

*Salk, Lee. *Preparing for Parenthood.* New York: David McKay Co., 1974.

Tanzer, Deborah. *Why Natural Childbirth?* New York: Doubleday, 1972.

Vellay, Pierre. *Childbirth with Confidence.* New York: MacMillan, 1969

Ward, Charlotte and Fred. *The Home Birth Book.* Washington, D.C.: Inscape, 1976.

In the course of research, I also referred to countless professional journals, many of which are listed in the preceding footnotes.

*Especially recommended for expectant mothers and fathers.

Index

Notes

Notes

Notes

Notes

Notes

Notes

About the author

Childbirth educator Valmai Howe Elkins was born in Australia in 1947 and is a graduate of the Melbourne School of Physiotherapy. Since 1967, she has lived in Canada, teaching thousands of couples her own version of Prepared Childbirth — which she has dubbed UPC. Director of the obstetrical program at McGill University's School of Physical and Occupational Therapy, she has written articles for various Canadian publications. Her frequent lectures, radio and television appearances have helped bring changes in childbirth to many North American and Australian communities. In 1978, she set up the first Birth Room program in Canada at the Sir Mortimer B. Davis Jewish General Hospital in Montreal. She is married to David Elkins, who coached the birth of their daughter Tilke in 1973.